The Ethical Risks of Professional Boundaries, When to Say Whoa, When to Say No

R. Dean White DDS MS
James C "Jes" Montgomery MD

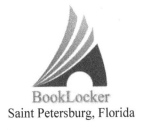

BookLocker
Saint Petersburg, Florida

Print ISBN: 978-1-64719-794-0
Ebook ISBN: 978-1-64719-795-7

Published by BookLocker.com, Inc., St. Petersburg, Florida.

Printed on acid-free paper.

BookLocker.com, Inc.
2021

First Edition

Library of Congress Cataloguing in Publication Data
White DDS MS, R. Dean and Montgomery MD, James C "Jes"
The Ethical Risks of Professional Boundaries, When to Say Whoa, When to Say No by R. Dean White DDS MS and James C "Jes" Montgomery MD
Library of Congress Control Number: 2021919168

DISCLAIMER

This book details the authors' personal and professional experiences with and opinions about the ethical risks of professional boundaries. The authors are not licensed ethicists.

The authors and publisher are providing this book and its contents on an "as is" basis and make no representations or warranties of any kind with respect to this book or its contents. The authors and publisher disclaim all such representations and warranties, including for example warranties of merchantability and psychological advice for a particular purpose. In addition, the author and publisher do not represent or warrant that the information accessible via this book is accurate, complete or current.

The statements made about products and services have not been evaluated by the U.S. government. Please consult with your own legal, accounting, medical, or other licensed professional regarding the suggestions and recommendations made in this book.

Except as specifically stated in this book, neither the author or publisher, nor any authors, contributors, or other representatives will be liable for damages arising out of or in connection with the use of this book. This is a comprehensive limitation of liability that applies to all damages of any kind, including (without limitation) compensatory; direct, indirect or consequential damages; loss of data, income or profit; loss of or damage to property and claims of third parties.

You understand that this book is not intended as a substitute for consultation with a licensed medical, legal or accounting professional. Before you begin any change your lifestyle in any way, you will consult a licensed professional to ensure that you are doing what's best for your situation.

This book provides content related to professional boundaries. As such, use of this book implies your acceptance of this disclaimer.

Table of Contents

Foreword ix

R Dean White DDS MS xv

James C. "Jes" Montgomery, MD xvii

Introduction 1

Chapter 1: Boundary Crossings and Violations 7

History and Research of Violations 10
No Provider Is Immune 14

Chapter 2: The Importance of The Provider's
Family Systems in the Formation of Appropriate
Boundaries 23

Creating Self-Awareness 24
Predispositions to Dysfunction 26
Genesis of Boundary Violations 26
Family Systems: Rules and Roles 28
Attachment Templates and Theories 34
Suggested Further Reading: 39

Chapter 3: The Road to Boundary Violations 41

Success, Power, and Distance 43
The Consequences of Medical Training and Career
Development 45

Chapter 4: The Influence of Empathy 69

The Importance and Benefits of Empathy 69
Acceptance and Evolution of Empathy in Healthcare 71

Empathy Defined 72

The Neuroscience of Empathy 73

Active Listening and Empathy 77

Achieving the Correct Balance 79

The Endgame of Empathy 83

Chapter 5: The Ethics of it All 87

How Ethics Applies to Medicine 91

Ethics and Romance 95

Chapter 6: Healthy Sexual Boundaries 99

The Sexual Journey 99

Is Sex the End of The Sexual Journey? 101

Masculinity, Femininity, and Vulnerability 104

Nonverbal Parts of Sexuality 106

Chapter 7: Separating the Problems from the
      Issues with Sexual Boundary Violations 109

When Does Behavior Become Problematic? 110

What Happens When Boundaries are Broken by
      Problematic Behavior? 112

Boundary Crossings and Boundary Transgressions 114

Assessment and treatment 116

Healthy Boundaries Help Define Healthy Sexuality and
      Behavior 118

The "Problem Patient" is Not the Issue 122

Redirecting Confusing Messages 123

Patients' Rights 126

Chapter 8: Electronic Media: Positives and Negatives .. 129

Social Media as a Tool 130

Pause Before You Post 135

Chapter 9: Long Term Strategies 141

Keeping stress and burnout at bay 142

Professional strategies to keep boundaries in check 145

Chapter 10: Potholes and Pearls 153

Foreword

In the fall of 2015, I found myself sitting around a U-shaped table in an intimate room on a hilltop in Argyle, Texas. I was joined by 9 other licensed professionals. Most of us present were physicians, but a nurse, lawyer and CEO rounded out our group. The majority of the attendees had been compelled by their respective licensing boards to attend the course entitled "Maintaining Proper Boundaries," a quarterly Continuing Medical Education presentation. The course is planned and implemented in accordance with the Essential Areas and Policies of the Accreditation Council for Continuing Medical Education through the joint providership of the University of Texas Southwestern Medical Center and the Santé Center for Healing.

To look around the room, one might think the group members were preparing for their collective execution. Expressions were grim. The continental breakfast buffet had barely been touched. If eye contact was made, it was brief and accompanied by a sheepish smile before quickly looking away. It was obvious that nobody was happy to be there.

Personally, I had enrolled in the course as part of my onboarding to practice at Santé. As a young mother with a baby and toddler at home, I was looking forward to switching from the hectic pace of a hospital environment to the more relaxed pace of working at a residential addiction treatment center. But this was not just any treatment center. Having lived and practiced in the Dallas-Fort Worth area for over a decade, I was familiar with Santé's remarkable reputation and was thrilled to join the treatment team. As a psychiatrist, addictionologist, and eating disorder specialist, I was well equipped to treat the majority of Santé's patients. There were, however, a few areas in which Santé specializes that I had received little to no education on in medical school and residency: problematic sexual behavior, sex addiction and boundaries. Ten years as a practicing physician, yet this would be my first formal course on these subjects.

The room was quiet in anticipation of the opening lecture. The attendees seemed embarrassed; the common thread was experiencing some level of professional reprimand. The reasons varied. Improper prescribing. An off-color remark to a coworker. A sexual relationship with a patient. Whatever the case, there were a million other places they would rather be than sitting in this particular room on this chilly autumn morning. Though the information shared could have prevented any of these situations mentioned above, regrettably so few "voluntarily" register for the course.

In sauntered Dr. White. He's a self-described old school country boy, an oral and maxillofacial surgeon who practiced in a time before #metoo was a thought, much less a movement. Dr. White has spent the majority of his career involved in medical staff governance. He has born personal witness to the dramatic and needed shift that has come into the workplace over the past few decades. Gone are the days a surgeon can curse at his team and throw tools on the floor in a fit of rage when things don't go his way. Gone are the days when an inappropriate joke or "harmless" flirtation with a co-worker is tolerated.

That morning Dr. White sat on the edge of one of the desks, relaxed and smiling. The thickness in the air lifted just a little bit. He acknowledged the fact that no one wanted to be there, and just by that small admission you could feel the mood lighten a bit more. His easy conversation and affable personality instantly put the room at ease.

After a brief introduction, he wasted no time in getting straight to the point, in asking the question that nobody wanted to talk about: *What brought you here?*

The amazing thing was, they told us. They were honest. They elaborated. As each person shared his or her own personal story, the shame of the others lifted little by little. In the span of less than an hour, they had revealed more about their lives to total strangers than they probably had to their closest friends.

It was on that same fortuitous day that I met Dr. Jes Montgomery for the first time. Having worked as a psychiatrist in the DFW area for several years, I was familiar with his name as Santé's previous medical director. We had shared several patients over the years, and by the way the patients spoke of him and his no-nonsense attitude towards addiction and recovery, I was expecting someone a little rougher around the edges. Yet Dr. Montgomery's edges were smooth. He is calm, soft-spoken, educated and eloquent. He has an air of intelligence and sophistication. Although large in physical stature, he is accommodating, approachable, almost shy.

In their instruction on boundaries, Dr. Montogomery and Dr. White create a safe space. There is no judgement. There is no punishment. There are just human beings coping with life on life's terms.

The homework on the first night of the boundaries course was to create a genogram, a family tree that maps out relationships, illnesses and addictions going back at least a couple of generations. There was a major shift that occurred in the group the following day- the day the genograms were discussed in small groups. Many of the professionals who attend the boundaries course are therapy-naïve. It was nothing short of miraculous to see the lightbulbs turn on. For the first time in their lives, they had gained some level of understanding of their relationship patterns, boundaries (or lack thereof) and how and why they came to be that way. Tears were shed. Grief was expressed. There was insight and appreciation. A freedom. A collective weight seemed to have been lifted from their shoulders, accompanied by a desire to change these newly discovered behavior patterns.

Having been through several boundaries courses over the past 5 years (specifically with my course faculty role), I can tell you that the mood shifts with each group. Most courses are bonding, cathartic experiences which leave the participants feeling whole and understood. A few are more like pulling teeth. The ego defenses are strong. The conversation is minimal. The disdain for the course and instructors is palpable.

Time has afforded me the opportunity to get to know both of the authors on a personal and professional level. I attend conferences with Dr. Montgomery and have traveled for speaking engagements with Dr. White. They have both been teaching on this important subject for years, and they can finally say they "wrote the book."

This is a book that needed to be written. It intersects with a critical time in the field of medicine. Burnout rates are at an all-time high. Depression and addictive disorders are on the rise. If we, as professionals, are unable to properly care for ourselves, how can we be expected to care for our patients? That self-care and awareness are at the core of maintaining healthy boundaries. The Ethical Risks of Professional Boundaries: When to Say Whoa, When to Say No provides an outline for identifying problematic thinking patterns, what proper boundaries look like, and the slippery slope behaviors than can eventually get us into trouble. As Dr. Montgomery likes to say, "It's not a problem... until it's a problem."

Let's prevent the problems with the wisdom and solutions contained within these pages.

Dr. Melissa Pennington
Medical Director, Santé Center for Healing
www.santecenter.com

R Dean White DDS MS

R Dean White has been involved in medical staff governance his entire career. He has served on virtually every medical staff committee and served as the Chief of the medical staff in 1999 and 2000 at Texas Health Harris Methodist HEB Hospital in the Dallas Ft Worth area. He served on the Board of Trustees for the same hospital for six years. He served, part time, as the Medical Staff Advisor from 2002 to 2011 and was responsible for medical staff orientations, leadership development, coaching and mentoring, behavioral event peer review and the physician health committee. He championed and helped implement the medical staff code of conduct in 2003.

Dr. White is the past president of the North Texas, Texas and Southwest Society of Oral and Maxillofacial Surgeons. He is a past president of The American Board of Oral and Maxillofacial Surgery. His clinical interests concentrated on temporomandibular joint surgical reconstruction and corrective jaw surgery. He had multiple peer reviewed publications as well as several book chapters to his credit before his retirement from oral and maxillofacial surgery in 2002.

Dr. White currently presents frequently and consults with medical staffs and their leadership as well as medical staff professionals on a state and national level. He serves on the faculty for Maintaining Proper Boundaries co sponsored by Santé Center for Healing and Southwestern Medical School which is presented quarterly. He has been a speaker for the Greeley Medical Staff Institute and the National Association of Medical Staff Services and the American College of Healthcare

Executives on several occasions. His topics include managing disruptive behavior and impairment, burnout and balance, the aging physician, leadership principles for physicians, medical staff boundaries, prescribing practices, ethics in a changed workplace and empathy training for the physician. He is the author of *A Practical Guide to Managing Disruptive and Impaired Physicians,* with Dr. Jon Burroughs , published by HCPro, December of 2010 and *Medical Staff Leadership Essentials: A Guide to Developing Leadership Skills and Recruiting the Next Generation*, HCPro, May, 2011 and *What the Hell Do I Do Now? A Professionals' Guide to a Meaningful Retirement*, published by Book Locker in 2012. He received his dental degree and oral and maxillofacial surgery training and master of science degree from the University of Texas Dental Branch in Houston Texas.

James C. "Jes" Montgomery, MD

Dr. Montgomery began his career in medicine as a Family Physician in 1983 after graduating from LSU School of Medicine in New Orleans in December 1979. Changes in the face of practice in Oil Industry laden South Louisiana led him to a transition to Addiction Medicine in 1987, receiving his certification in treating Addictions in 1987 by the American Medical Society on Alcohol and Other Drug Dependencies (AMSAODD), which became the America Society of Addiction Medicine (ASAM). He worked in Addiction Medicine until 1992, when he entered psychiatry residency at LSU Medical Center in New Orleans. Upon graduation, he moved to Dallas and began a private practice while working part-time positions with the Chemical Dependency Unit at the VAMC, in the Psychiatric Emergency Room and as Adjunct Faculty at the University of Texas Southwestern Medical Center. He also began a private practice of General Psychiatry. In 1996, he was the founding Medical Director at Sante Center for Healing in Argyle Texas, a residential treatment center which treated all addictions, but focused on healthcare professionals with addictive disorders and sexual boundary violations. Between 1995 and 1997, he worked with the Ross Institute for Trauma Treatment at Timberlawn Hospital and, in 1997, became the Medical Director at the Pride Unit, a program of Addiction Treatment for the LGBTQ population at Millwood Hospital. In 2003, he returned to Sante Center for Healing and transitioned into Medical Director, also participating in the "Maintaining Proper Boundaries Course" under the guidance of

Vanderbilt University and UTSW until 2011, when he assumed the psychiatric directorship of the Gentle Path Sexual Addiction Program at Pine Grove Behavioral Health and Addictions in Hattiesburg, MS until 2016, continuing as a consultant to the present. Dr. Montgomery had served two terms on the Board of the Society for the Advancement of Sexual Health and was awarded the Carnes Award for Achievement in Sexual Addiction in 2010. He was also awarded the President's Award for contribution to the field by the National Association for Lesbian and Gay Addiction Professionals, also in 2010. He has presented at numerous medical societies and conferences on topics related to boundaries, sexual health and problematic sexual behaviors over the years. He continues to provide input into psychosexual evaluation of healthcare providers for Pine Grove and directly to Physician Health Programs.

Introduction

The bond between the healer and the patient is unique. The provider is often considered all-knowing, incapable of making mistakes, and automatically worthy of a patient's trust. The patient can often feel vulnerable and afraid, seeking answers and relief. In many cases, the provider holds the patient's life in their hands. With such an imbalance of power, appropriate, well-established boundaries are critical to keeping the patient safe and the treatment beneficial. As we enter the unchartered waters of more government-driven and corporate medicine, it is paramount that the provider-patient relationship remains the foundation to the delivery of high-quality healthcare. Boundaries are delicate—they must not become barriers to good medicine and care. Still, they must be firmly in place to avoid harm.

Consider the boundaries between a healthcare provider and his or her patients to be a study in ethics, where the situation at hand often determines what is appropriate and what is not. In many situations, there is a marked distinction between what is right and what is wrong, but most boundary discussions occur within the gray zones of thought and logic. The critical fact is that the power belongs to the professional, and, for the most part, the vulnerability belongs to the patient. Healthcare professionals run the risk of forsaking our humanity if we adhere to strict boundaries that ignore empathy and common sense while establishing relationships with patients. All caregivers interact with patients or clients when they are most vulnerable, and the trust they place in us is sacred. It is important to honor this trust, both for the current interaction and for all patient interactions to follow. Once this trust is lost, it is very difficult to restore.

This book is designed to help all professionals who have fiduciary responsibility over others to provide safe and effective care by maintaining proper boundaries that protect both the patient and the caregiver. It is designed to help physicians, nurses, therapists, dentists, and counselors to formulate their own boundaries, keeping in mind that the letters after your name make you ultimately responsible for any violation of set boundaries. Both authors have extensive experience in teaching proper boundaries in small groups, classrooms, continuing education courses, and publications. We draw on our own experiences as clinicians and educators to present a practical guide on how to set and maintain proper boundaries.

The boundaries between an OB-Gyn and a patient will be markedly different than the boundaries between a priest and a couple he or she is counseling; therefore, boundary setting requires a deeper look than just what specialty is at hand. Professionals must understand themselves and their patients deeply to create and maintain appropriate boundaries.

What to Expect from this Book

This book will discuss boundaries and boundary violations, as well as what constitutes an acceptable boundary crossing versus a violation that can lead to the loss of one's professional license. Further, we will delve into the psychology of the highly educated professional to help explain why you are who you are and why you must be cognizant of your place in the caregiver-patient equation.

We also discuss the effect your family of origin and cultural background have on your own formulation of proper boundaries. Understanding how a childhood disrupted by addiction, illness, or instability, as well as family rules and roles can predict your future relationships, both personal and professional, is a critical step for any healthcare professional. Codependency, psychological attachment templates, and trauma play a role in your own vulnerability. Understanding these basic psychological principles will help you avoid the pitfalls inherent in the provider-patient relationship.

This book will also cover the history of empathy and its importance in the healthcare environment. When medicine began, practitioners were taught to be completely detached and unemotional, but over the last few years, the concept of empathy has resurged and is being measured and taught during residency and fellowship training programs. Empathy is fundamental to setting boundaries. We will explain how to achieve the correct balance of empathy and detachment, how to use concepts of emotional intelligence, and how to apologize when appropriate.

In this book, the power differential between caregiver and patient and the basic ethics of boundaries are explained, and we help identify factors that predispose certain caregivers to vague boundaries and who may be more prone to exceeding boundaries. Most caregivers are not thought to have any issues or vulnerabilities, but of course, that is not true. Caregivers are just as prone to mental, addictive, or physical illness as patients.

These are equal-opportunity diseases that do not skip the healthcare provider.

So often, we assume that the party that violated a boundary is the caregiver, but patients often cross or violate boundaries as well. Thus, we will illustrate techniques to help you avoid trouble with seductive patients, clients, or employees. We will also discuss the advancement of digital communication and social media and its huge influence on interpersonal relationships. Social media often blurs the definition of appropriate self-disclosure and confidentiality and, at times can cause the ultimate breakdown of healthy boundaries.

Sexuality, an important aspect of who we are, will be discussed as well. Denying one's own sexuality is not realistic, but if it is misused, it can lead to allegations of sexual harassment or hostile workplace environment. Such charges can lead to the loss of a professional's license. Understanding how a boundary crossing becomes sexual harassment is critical.

This book also covers long-term strategies of self-assessment, balance, thankfulness, and how to interact with your fiduciary regulatory body or board. We also include a discussion on how to formulate treatment plans to keep you within your boundaries and how to detect possible problems before they arise. The reader is provided with checklists reflecting personal inventories as tools for self-assessment.

Ultimately, as the professional in the room, you will set the boundaries that dictate how you manage your relationship with patients. It is incumbent that you set those boundaries with empathy and intelligence to protect both the patient and yourself. All healthcare providers should know themselves better, as well as the principles of ethics and boundaries. Doing so ensures you are doing everything within your power to treat patients without doing harm.

Chapter 1:
Boundary Crossings and Violations

We are all human, and for the most part, we are complex social beings. This is a good thing. We are all products of nature and nurture. We have different ethnicities, cultures, belief systems, sexual orientations, degrees of intelligence and education, and personalities. We do not and should not automatically shed everything that makes us unique when we become licensed to provide healthcare, therapy, or counseling services to our fellow human beings. However, keeping these human strengths and weaknesses apart from our professional roles is what maintaining proper boundaries is all about. At its core, this is not a simple task.

In the healthcare setting, boundaries are defined as the expected and accepted psychological and social distance between practitioners and patients. Boundaries are defined by ethics, culture, morality, and law. It is often difficult to make a clear distinction between where your boundary ends and where a patient's or client's boundary begins.[1] The Texas Medical Association states that boundaries are "mutually understood, unspoken physical and emotional limits of the professional relationship between a patient and the physician or student, or the supervisor and student."[2]

---

[1] Gutheil T.G. and Simon, R.I. (2002) Non-sexual boundary crossings and violations: The ethical dimension. *Psychiatric Clin N Am*, 25, 585–92.
[2] Committee on Physician Health and Rehabilitation, Texas Medical Association. (2012). Challenges of Professional Boundaries (for Medical Students).

Jane Barton, a noted author and speaker on "compassion fatigue" for the caregiver, particularly in palliative care environments, defines boundaries as "the limits that protect the space between the professional's power and the patient's vulnerability."[3] Boundaries are fluid, rarely well-defined, nearly always situational, and prone to misinterpretation. There are non-sexual boundary crossings and violations and there are sexual boundary crossings and violations; however, the former often leads to the latter, making an in-depth knowledge of crossings and violations a critical tool for all caregivers.

Most boundary crossings could be considered normal social interactions. Complimenting someone else's attire, inquiring about his or her family, using first names or nicknames, and patting someone on the shoulder to comfort or reassure are all examples of boundary crossings. These small acts seem innocent enough, yet, all of these examples could signal the potential for future boundary violations if nonverbal communication is considered. Physical proximity, eye contact, speech volume and tone of voice during any of these examples could convey a potential boundary violation.

It takes two to communicate, and we may not be able to discern what the other person is thinking, feeling, or trying to convey. Humans take all their social clues—what is heard, seen, and felt—and create a guess of the other person's intentions and what he or she is trying to convey (i.e., where the other person is "coming from"). As the professional in the equation, it is your responsibility to communicate without harm and with your

---

[3] Barton, J. Professional Boundaries: Discerning a line in the sand. Life Quality Institute.

patient's best interest at heart. Many non-sexual crossings are everyday occurrences in our practices. Having patients who are friends, seeing family or staff members as patients, entering in a business venture with a patient, forwarding an inappropriate email, liking a patient's social media status update, or telling a joke are all examples of crossings. Standing too close to someone while speaking or remaining in a standing position when the other person is seated are also examples of crossings. Excessive cologne or perfume can be a crossing bordering on a violation as well. The list is endless.

Sexual crossings are determined by the intent and context. The margin of error here is much too narrow for most of us to navigate effectively. The difference between patting someone's shoulder for comfort and squeezing it is not all that great, nor is the difference between a pat on the knee versus a hand resting on the knee, or the sideways upper-body hug versus the full-frontal hug, but they are all examples of boundary crossings teetering on the edge of violation. Obviously, sexual touching or a sexual relationship with a patient or client is the ultimate breakdown of a professional boundary and in most locales is not only viewed as unethical, but also illegal. There is no place for mutual consent because the patient is never in a position to consent; the innate power differential between professional and patient or client keeps the patient/client too vulnerable to make clear and appropriate decisions.

History and Research of Violations

One would think that everyone would agree that sexual contact between a practitioner and a patient would be at the least unethical and, for the most part, illegal. After all, beginning in 4th century B.C., the Hippocratic Oath stated an unequivocal position on the matter: "Whatever houses that I may visit, I will come for the benefit of the sick, remaining free of all intentional injustice, of all mischief and in particular of sexual relationships whether male or female persons, be they free or slaves." However, the American Medical Association's Council on Ethical and Judicial affairs statement in 1990 appears to address the same conundrum but curiously uses the pesky word "may:"

> *Sexual contact which occurs concurrent with the physician-patient relationship constitutes sexual misconduct. Sexual or romantic interactions between physicians and patients detract from the goals of the physician-patient relationship, <u>may</u> exploit the vulnerability of the patient, <u>may</u> obscure the physician's objective judgment concerning the patient's health care, and <u>may</u> ultimately be detrimental to the patient's wellbeing.* [emphasis added]

Unfortunately, literature on the topic of sexual boundary violations has been written mostly by psychiatrists discussing other psychiatrists. The literature concerning sexual boundaries written by physicians is scarce, and the literature for other healthcare professions is practically non-existent. The clergy has a few references on the issue, but not many. In recent years, the public press has certainly been diligent in reporting current and past abuses of pastoral and celebrity power. So, what can we learn from this?

A quick look at the literature that does exist highlights that the problem doesn't just lie within one specialty, gender, or level of education. It also indicates that what seems inappropriate to some seems perfectly acceptable to others.

The prevalence of inappropriate physician-patient contact was described in an article by Gartrell.[4] In 1992, researchers sent an anonymous survey of four questions to 10,000 family practitioners, internists, obstetrician-gynecologists, and surgeons.

In total, 1,891 surveys were answered and sent back. Nine percent of the respondents admitted to having sexual contact with one or more current patients. Of those 9%, 89% were male physicians having relations with female patients. The survey respondents were also asked:

1. Is it professionally acceptable to have sexual contact with a current patient?
2. Is it professionally acceptable for a physician to have sexual contact with a patient still taking medication prescribed by that physician?
3. Is it professionally acceptable to have sexual contact with a patient whose treatment has stopped and who has been referred to another physician?
4. Do you favor state licensing boards prohibiting physician-patient sexual contact?

---

[4] Gartrell, N.K., Milliken, N., et al. (1992). Physician-patient sexual contact-prevalence and problems. *West J Med, 157*, 139–143.

Amazingly, 63% of the total number of respondents thought the contact was "almost always" harmful to the patients. Although the vast majority of respondents (94%) opposed sexual contact with current patients, that figure leaves 6% who would appear to approve. That leaves about 113 professionals who did not oppose sexual contact with patients. When asked whether participants found it professionally acceptable to become the physician of a current or former sexual partner—being a romantic or sexual partner first, then a patient—39% said yes. Out of this 39%, men (41%) were more likely than women (26%) to consider it acceptable.

Importantly, 63% (or 1,173) of the respondents thought it was acceptable to have a romantic or sexual relationship after the professional patient-provider relationship had ceased. The research regarding having a romantic or sexual relationship with a former patient—having a professional relationship before a romantic or sexual one—led researchers to adopt the Ontario Task Force's recommendation[5] that at least two years must have elapsed since the last episode of patient care, with no social contact in the interim, to make a sexual relationship acceptable between a physician and patient. The problematic portion of this conclusion, however, is that the power differential has not necessarily disappeared after two years. Context here might serve as crucial guidance. What if the patient-provider relationship consisted of a one-time dermatology appointment or an emergency appendectomy?

---

[5] McPhedran M., Armstrong H., Edney R., et al. (1991). The Preliminary Report of the Task Force on Sexual Abuse of Patients, Toronto, Ontario, College of Physicians and Surgeons of Ontario.

These instances create a much different relationship than a long-term professional relationship a primary care provider or psychiatrist might have with a patient. Still, the power differential does not dilute with time for most relationships. And if, for instance, a male or female practitioner has had boundary issues in the past, then that individual would be wise to avoid all contact with former patients. Sometimes, others' perception becomes reality. Sometimes what appears innocent could be construed as a violation. If the physician has had a past transgression or allegation, then he or she may be judged by different standards than those who have not had this experience. Thus, a perception becomes a reality for the healthcare professional, even if her or she did nothing wrong. A healthcare professional with a past has to be more vigilant and aware of boundaries.

An excellent article by Brooks[6] studies the breadth and depth of boundary violations within healthcare by surveying Colorado physicians who had been referred to the state physician health program between 1986 and 2005. Physician health programs are organized by hospital staff or state societies to advocate, support, and monitor professionals whose personal issues affect their professional performance, including boundary issues. Referrals can be mandatory or voluntary. The sample size consisted of 1,133 physician who had been referred for a myriad of reasons, including substance abuse, mood disorders, stress, and boundary violations. There were 120

---

[6] Brooks, E., Gendel, M.H, et al. (2012). Physician Boundary Violations in a Physician Health Program: A 19 Year review. *J Am Acad Psychiatry Law, 40,* 59–66.

physicians referred specifically for boundary violations. The vast majority of these physicians (93%) were men between the ages of 40 and 49; 63% of the offenders were married. A variety of specialties were represented: 22% were psychiatrists, 18% were family practitioners, 15% were internists, and 8% were Ob-Gyns (the other 37% comprised a variety of specialties). Thirty percent of the 120 physicians with boundary issues had a personal history of physical or sexual abuse.

Researchers found that the most common boundary violations were prescribing violations (25%), followed by 14% of physicians having sexual relations with a former patient, and 11% having sexual relationships with a current patient. Researchers also reported that physicians who were referred to the physician health program for inappropriate prescribing and sexual harassment (defined as harassment that is sexual in nature but does not involve touching or contact, such as inappropriate language or creating a hostile work environment) had a tendency to elevate the violations to actual sexual relationships with current or former patients. The good news is that upon completing the program, which provides physicians with contracts that usually hold them accountable for their transgressions (for example, loss of medical license), 88% of the physicians had no further boundary transgressions.

No Provider Is Immune

All practitioners have vulnerabilities. This applies to some more than others. The practitioner who has a history of healthy, long-term relationships, grew up in a positive and healthy family environment, has developed a secure attachment template, and is healthy from a mental, social, and psychological standpoint may be in a better position to have broader and more lenient boundaries. A professional with prior boundary violations or complaints, or a background and history that indicates that person is a potential boundary violator will need tighter and more confined boundaries. Some might see this as an unfair protocol, but to continue to provide healthcare services, professionals are responsible for staying on the correct side of the boundary line. We have the power; thus, we have the responsibility. Keep in mind that boundary violations negatively affect the trust between professionals, patients, and colleagues, creating breaks that are incredibly difficult to mend.

The following clinical scenarios illustrate the differences between boundary crossings and violations. Many readers will find nothing wrong or unethical with most of them. However, perhaps after reading this book and considering all the different factors that influence patients, readers will see a potential for them to be boundary crossings, if not violations. As you read them consider the following questions:

1. Is this a boundary crossing or a violation?
2. Whose needs are being met?
3. What could have been done differently?
4. Can you find yourself in any of these scenarios?

Scenario A

A 40-year-old single female dermatologist has been seeing a 37-year-old male for contact dermatitis for the last two years. They see each other at a mutual friend's New Year's Eve party and start to discuss common interests of modern art. At his next appointment, he brings her a coffee table book from the Guggenheim Museum as a gift for helping him with his dermatologic problems. She is flattered. She accepts the gift and places it in her waiting room.

Scenario B

A baby-boomer-aged dentist is referred a well-known rock star from the 1980s for a consultation for a dental implant. At the initial appointment, the patient brings in signed CDs for the dentist and all his staff members. Everyone is excited. The dentist instructs his front office appointment clerk to give the special patient the last appointment of the week so that he wouldn't be bothered by other patients.

Scenario C

A female family therapist has a thriving practice in a moderately sized Midwestern town. Since the inception of her practice, she would call selected clients to check on them before the weekend to be sure they were doing okay. When questioned by her staff whether this was appropriate, she responds, "It keeps me from being called over the weekend, and I can head off any problems before they develop."

Scenario D

The mother of a cardiothoracic surgeon is referred to her son by a university cardiologist for coronary bypass surgery. Her son is the chair of the department and heads a large heart team of attendings, fellows, and residents. His mother is elated that her son is willing to take care of her. After all, she knows "he is the very best."

Scenario E

A young family practitioner in a small rural town in east Texas is starting to develop his practice. His empathy and listening skills are commendable. As each staff member joins his team, they have their medical records transferred to their new employer so that he can be their physician. It would seem a betrayal for them to stay with the other family practice in town, and he is grateful for the confidence they have in him.

Scenario F

A female psychiatrist has an attractive younger female patient that continues to demand just a little more time at each appointment. The patient is always asking questions of the psychiatrist's personal life and requests a hug at the end of each session. The psychiatrist has agreed to meet the patient for lunch after her next appointment in an attempt to change this behavior.

Scenario G

An internist volunteers at a local charity clinic once a week in a nearby city. All of the patients are indigent, and many don't appear to have the means to follow up with his instructions or prescriptions. One day, the social worker that was assigned to him was unavailable to help with the proper forms and referrals for a 67-year-old hypertensive patient who needed help obtaining an important prescription. The patient was frustrated, and so was the internist, so he gave her $20.00 to use at the local Wal-Mart to have the prescription filled.

Scenario H

A nurse practitioner (NP) from a large internal medicine clinic is away on vacation with her family in the mountains close to where she practices. The first morning of the week-long vacation, one of her daughters has what appears to be an acute maxillary sinus infection. The NP gives her daughter some Augmentin samples she had with her, as well as some over-the-counter antihistamines and decongestants. The next morning, the daughter is complaining of significant infraorbital pain. Her mother gives her hydrocodone tablets to help with the pain.

Scenario I

One of the extra benefits of working for a busy cosmetic facial plastic surgeon is the office camaraderie. They celebrate office birthdays with after-hours cocktails every month. The surgeon's annual bonus for employees is a trip to Cancun for an extended weekend with him and his wife. Everyone is on a first-name basis. The surgeon has also operated on most of his employees to provide what he calls "walking advertisements."

Scenario J

A hospice nurse has become quite attached to her elderly patient, Emma, and Emma's family. Emma reminds the nurse of her grandmother who passed away last year. The nurse collects Fostoria antique glassware, and the family has a large collection of the same glassware that the nurse noticed in the family home. Emma's family has decided to give it all to the nurse in appreciation for her compassionate care of their mother.

Scenario K

Dr. Lee, an orthodontist, has an active Facebook page and twitter accounts. She encourages all of her patients to "friend" her and follow her on Twitter. She routinely posts her social activities, trips, and purchases. Her patients love her for including them in her life. Through this social media connection, her practice is growing by leaps and bounds secondary to patient referrals.

Which of these scenarios did you find troubling? Do you consider any of them boundary violations? Which do you think have the potential to cause trouble for the practitioner and/or patient down the road? Do any of these scenarios seem innocent or non-problematic?

That providers should avoid empathetic interaction with patients to provide healthcare isn't what should be inferred from these scenarios. Rather, this exercise was to highlight that boundaries are situational and contextual. All healthcare professionals cross boundaries daily, and some providers truly benefit from the physician-patient relationship. Thus, for the most part, this has a positive effect on patients' care and outcomes. Providers, of course, can be kind and caring human beings. We all would benefit from knowing each other better. That might involve a hug, a pat on the shoulder, conversations about loved ones, etc. But it is also easy to see which of these scenarios could constitute boundary violations if not moderated.

The point of keeping boundaries is to not lose sight of our primary goal as healthcare providers, which is to help the patient. Boundaries are critical to this goal, but if your intent is well placed, crossing the boundary will more than likely be beneficial to both of you.

Take the case of a true story published in *The Man with the Iron Tattoo* by John Castaldo, MD, and Lawrence Levitt, MD, both neurologists.[7] The story is that of an elderly female patient with cognitive decline of unknown origin. Dr. Levitt is a young neurology resident who discovers that the decline is the result of an anti-diuretic hormone. During the patient's stay, her husband will not leave her bedside. He sleeps in his clothes on a cot the entire time she is in the hospital and appears to not have money for a hotel. Dr. Levitt recounts the story of the loyal husband to his wife, who suggests having the husband over for dinner. Dr. Levitt invites the husband and they enjoy a dinner filled with conversation. The husband is quite pleased to be included in dinner. The patient improves and is discharged.

A few days later, the CEO of the hospital calls Dr. Levitt to his office to inform him that his dinner guest was the wealthy owner of a large chemical company and has pledged $1 million to the hospital. This man later donates even more to underwrite a neurology center that both physicians work at for the next 30 years. This extraordinary experience leads the authors to urge doctors to "look around and notice people who seem anxious,

---

[7] J Castaldo, L Levitt, The Man with the Iron Tattoo, BenBella Books, Dallas, 2006

frightened or lonely... to sit down, take the time to hear what matters to them."

In this chapter, you have learned that:

- Boundaries are defined as the expected and accepted psychological and social distance between professionals and patient
- Boundaries protect the space between the professional's power and the patient's vulnerability
- Boundary crossings can easily slide into boundary violations
- Context is critical in determining whether a situation crosses or violates boundaries
- The professional is always responsible for maintaining appropriate boundaries
- No professional or provider is immune from making mistakes or crossing boundaries occasionally

Chapter 2:
The Importance of The Provider's Family Systems in the Formation of Appropriate Boundaries

This book aims to define the professional relationship between two people: the healthcare provider and whoever he or she interacts with in the professional setting. People with whom the provider interacts can include patients or clients or the patient/clients' families; the office or hospital staff; or even the provider's own family. Both parties bring vulnerabilities to the relationship equation, and this equation is not always balanced.

Many medical schools have been slow to provide education relating to boundary issues. Therefore, practitioners may go into practice unaware of patients' vulnerabilities or their own. In fact, almost 60% of the respondents of Gartrell's survey (see Chapter 1) stated that the issue of boundaries and sexual contact had not been discussed during their medical training.

In fact, the boundary courses that the authors teach at the Sante Center for Healing and the University of Texas Southwestern Medical Center are often populated by psychiatrists and mental health professionals who one might think would have a better understanding of relationship boundaries than other practitioners. Given that a good number of mental health professionals participate in the courses suggests that all healthcare professionals would likely benefit from a review of boundaries—how they are formed, and how each individual might be likely to cross them in an inappropriate, unethical, or unprofessional manner.

Creating Self-Awareness

Understanding and accepting that there is a psychology and theory behind what we do and why we do it is critical to addressing boundary violation risk and relationships in general. It is also important to understand how our childhoods and past experiences affect our current actions. However, before we can learn what makes us vulnerable to relationship pitfalls in our professional lives, we *must* accept that psychological theories apply to everyone. Although many people (healthcare professionals in particular) claim to accept this idea broadly, accepting it personally may be easier said than done. For example, there are still a large number of people who believe addiction is a moral failing even though research proves that addiction is a physiological, chemically induced trigger. Many professionals and patients are hesitant to acknowledge that they have vulnerabilities. Admitting to vulnerability leaves one feeling vulnerable—a state many of us often go to great lengths to avoid.

The goal of this chapter is to explore human vulnerabilities based on family background and what are known as "attachment templates," a discipline that evaluates the mother-child relationship as it relates to child development and adult behavior. Every practitioner will have different and varied boundaries depending on the patient, family member, or staff member in question. Boundary lines will also shift based on context and situation. The hope is that we can determine our boundaries based on our own personal history and that of our patients. It is important to recognize that each individual is a combination of past experiences and innate character and personality traits, including us as professionals. Therefore, it may be necessary to ask yourself some difficult questions before accepting a patient or client for treatment.

Practicing medicine with self-awareness may seem simple, such as thinking twice before making an offhand comment to a staff member or prescribing medication for one of your own family members. But even with a heightened sense of self-awareness, many situations are much more nuanced and difficult to navigate. For example, an off-hand comment directed at a person without a traumatic history of sexual abuse might have no consequences; however, the same comment might set off or deeply affect a patient who does have a traumatic history of sexual abuse. Prescribing a narcotic for chronic back pain might be legitimate medical care for one patient but might violate boundaries if that patient is a friend with a family history of narcotic abuse. Conversely, if *your* family has a history of narcotic abuse, you may be less likely to prescribe them to someone who might legitimately need it. Similarly, if you are recently single, you might find yourself making inappropriate comments to or flirting with patients. Conversely, you might find a patient's flirtatious mood unsettling if you have gone through a recent difficult break-up. Understand and recognize the power that self-awareness has toward guiding your behavior around patients.

Predispositions to Dysfunction

Of course, we cannot choose our parents, and we did not determine how we were nurtured as children or adolescents; regardless, these experiences can have a profound effect on the physician-patient relationship. It is beyond the scope of this book to explore all the theories of family systems and attachment templates, but an overview will help you better understand who you are and your vulnerabilities such that you can more successfully avoid boundary violations. Your family of origin may predispose you to addiction, compulsivity, co-dependency, lack of self-esteem, and relationship and communication difficulties, to name a few. It is critical to be patently honest with yourself as you reflect on your family of origin and its degree of function or dysfunction. Denial does not help. Dysfunctional families many times produce dysfunctional adults.

If you recognize your past or your family in the following sections, then you may be at a higher risk for boundary violations or allegations of sexual misconduct. Knowledge is power; understanding where you stand will put in place taller and tighter boundaries than those who may come from more stable and functional backgrounds. Rather than become upset or defensive about this truth, recognize that boundaries are individual and situational; not everyone fits in the same box.

Genesis of Boundary Violations

Boundary violations that lead to sexual misconduct within the professional relationship could stem from a lack of knowledge of what is appropriate behavior. Personality characteristics, external stressors, addiction, compulsivity, and other mental or emotional disorders all probably contribute to any boundary violation. A study by Samenow and Yabiku provides compelling evidence that a practitioner's family of origin can predispose him or her to violate professional boundaries.[8]

The article, published in 2011, studied 613 physicians who were referred to a course on maintaining proper boundaries at the Sante Center for Healing and the University of Texas Southwestern Medical Center (Both authors of the book serve as faculty for these courses.). Most participants were referred by medical or dental boards for sexual misconduct allegations that involved everything from inappropriate comments or jokes to affairs with staff or colleagues to sexual violations with current patients. Although technically participants are attending the course voluntarily, their medical licenses and/or hospital privileges were at stake. Controls for the study were physicians who audited the course and did not have any allegations of sexual misconduct. Physicians who were referred were predominately male, white, married, and middle-aged. They represented a variety of specialties, including internists and family practitioners (37%), psychiatrists (10%), and obstetrician/gynecologists (7%). The remaining percentage represented a variety of specialties. Researchers studied the participants' families of origin, which were determined by a

---

[8] CP Samenow, ST Yabiku, et al. (2011). The Role of Family of Origin in Physicians Referred to a CME Course, Springer Science and Business Media.

FACES II survey, a validated and reliable measure of family dynamics. The tool measures family satisfaction by using two dimensions of family dynamics: (1) flexibility, ranging from too flexible (chaotic) to not flexible enough (rigid); and (2) cohesion, ranging from too close (enmeshed) to not close enough (disengaged). About 32% of the attendees described having been raised in families that were "balanced," while 30% fell midrange. The largest percentage (38%) had family patterns that fell into the "extreme" family, the group with the unhealthiest family structure. It was interesting to note that 91% in the "extreme" category described their families as disengaged and rigid.

A brief explanation of family systems helps identify vulnerability in the provider and patient/client (or whoever the professional interacts with in his or her professional role) and why some of us are predisposed to violating professional boundaries. Virginia Satir was a leading proponent of the influential concept that the family of origin has a strong influence on child development and subsequent adult behavior.[9] Two of her major theories—on family rules and family roles— lead to our discussion at hand.

Family Systems: Rules and Roles

Your family of origin has a significant influence on your attitudes and behaviors as an adult. Families are systems and, as such, seek an equilibrium or balance. This balance becomes off kilter when families exhibit inappropriate roles, overly

---

[9] V Satir, (1987). Conjoint Family Therapy, *Science and Behavior*

restrictive rules, and unrealistic expectations. When these poor habits are put into motion, the family members' needs are not met, and dysfunction occurs.

A healthy family system is described as nurturing and safe. The rules are clear, reasonable, and consistently enforced. Emotions are responded to appropriately. This system is flexible, accommodates change, and accepts diversity. It is predictable, consistent, and allows spontaneity when it arises. Most importantly, the balanced family system is respectful, using open communication that allows everyone to express his or her individual feelings without fear or recrimination.

The unhealthy family system is often so rigid that the members are not allowed to function outside of their assigned roles. The rules are inconsistent, as are consequences. The unhealthy family system is unpredictable, falling into a pattern of chaos followed by more rigidity when the family attempts to control the chaos (which happens randomly and non-routinely). This family has spoken and unspoken rules that dictate and guide the group's interactions, including what is talked about, how conflict is dealt with, and how the family responds to emotions and feelings. This is a top-down system, where "do as I say, not as I do" rules apply. Unfortunately, this type of mentality is found when the parents adhere to a strong military-like code, are overly legalistic in their religious beliefs, or have family secrets that they feel must be kept from the outside world. The end result for a child in a dysfunctional family is low self-esteem and defensive behavior that is later exhibited in adulthood.

In his book *Bradshaw on: The Family: A New Way of Creating Solid Self-Esteem,* author and speaker John Bradshaw defines dysfunctional families as a patriarchal method of keeping children in place by shaming and punishment. The result is low self-esteem. He states that "any family can become dysfunctional during times of extreme stress or anxiety. Strong families are characterized by high levels of parental maturity, having better and more flexible coping skills. Because such families have better coping strategies, they reduce their stress and limit the time [duration] of family dysfunction." He later writes that "Healthy families are characterized by the level of self-esteem that each parent has achieved. The ability to self-differentiate reduces the amount of reaction and irrational behavior of the family." Satir, in her book *People Makers* (1972), describes families that communicate poorly or not at all as dysfunctional as well. In other words, families that do not communicate with each other, and/or are ambiguous or dishonest, tend to produce children with low self-esteem, which in turn triggers maladaptive responses as adults.

An adult's response to growing up in a dysfunctional family can include codependence, substance abuse, inappropriate expectations, poor communication skills, etc. Not only are family systems responsible for an adult's dysfunctional behavior, but also for the moral, ethical, and spiritual education and modeling for their own children, meaning that the dysfunction can be passed down to the next generation.

Family Roles

Satir theorizes that each member in a dysfunctional family takes on a different role as a communicator. Family roles attempt to stabilize the family system by creating consistency and structure, but don't actually solve any of the underlying dysfunction. In a dysfunctional family, the rigid roles family members assume replace the honest and open communication that is found in a healthy family system in which roles are fluid. We all probably take on these roles at some time during our development in childhood. However, these roles should not be the primary core of our personality. The role an individual had as a child/adolescent within a dysfunctional family may define who that person is today and how he or she approaches the caregiver/patient relationship as well as all other professional relationships.

The definitions of Satir's roles have changed over time, but the premise remains. Many healthcare providers may have played the role of the **hero**, or the responsible child of the family. He or she is independent, overachieving, organized, self-disciplined, goal-oriented, and a leader. While these are positive characteristics, the hero feels a strong desire to keep their feelings hidden. They are perfectionists and may lack the ability to follow others or be spontaneous. The hero has a strong desire to control his or her environment or the people around them.

The **clown**, or mascot, of the family is funny, flexible, and able to relieve family and personal stress by his or her actions. Essentially, they are skilled at lightening the mood. The clown, however, continually seeks attention. Clowns use their sense of humor to hide emotions, may be immature, and can be poor decision makers.

The **scapegoat**, or drama queen, is creative and funny, can show emotions and can lead; however, he or she may express emotions inappropriately, and can be self-destructive and irresponsible. Scapegoats tend to have social problems and can be defiant. They are often underachievers.

The **lost child**, or adjuster, is independent, flexible, able to follow others, and has an easygoing attitude. This type is quiet and can entertain him- or herself easily. People in this role are often unable to initiate or stand up for themselves. They are fearful of making decisions, lack direction, and are lonely.

The **caretaker**, or people-pleaser, role also fits many healthcare professionals. People in this role are caring, compassionate, and empathetic, with good listening skills. They are sensitive, effective, and good team players. The challenges of this role are that they deny personal needs and have a high tolerance for inappropriate behavior. They fear conflict, can be anxious and fearful, and they become resentful when their care for others is not recognized or praised.

Satir describes healthy families as flexible and open. They communicate easily and solve problems together, as a family. Healthy families understand that we all will fail at times, but they respond with grace and unconditional love when someone in the family fails. Bradshaw describes a functional family as "the healthy soil of which individuals can become mature adults." A healthy family is a survival and growth unit; it provides for the emotional needs of its members. These needs include a balance between autonomy and dependency, as well as social and sexual training. A healthy family provides for growth and development of each member, including the parents, and is where solid self-esteem building takes place. The family is the matrix in which the children's moral values are formed.

Family Rules

Family rules can be spoken and unspoken and play a central part in the development of the child and functioning of the family. Some examples of these spoken or unspoken rules are:

- "Do as I say, not as I do."
- "Children are to be seen, not heard."
- "Your father or mother does not have an alcohol/gambling/drug problem."
- "Always be good, always be perfect."
- "It is not okay to talk about problems or show any emotion."
- "Big boys don't cry."
- "If you control things and people, you will be safe."

When these spoken or unspoken rules exist in the family, there is no openness or honesty. All interactions are tainted with the effort of keeping the illusion that the family is healthy and normal. For example, if your family of origin one or two generations removed, such as your parents or grandparents, shows addiction and compulsivity involving work, alcohol, drugs, gambling, or sex, then there may be reason for concern. Most families of alcoholics are dysfunctional and are severely enmeshed. Often, children are entrapped and entangled as they try to satisfy the needs of both parents by trying to keep a balance in the family and the outward appearance that all is right with the world. The boundaries between parent and child are porous and overrun, creating a loss in which the child does not get to be a child. This type of family behavior is a form of abandonment.

In families with these rules, all the roles are rigid and predetermined by the system or the parents. If you were raised in a strict military or overly religious family, then there may also be reasons for self-assessment and discussion. Often, these families include at least one parent who expects the children to follow a code (religious or otherwise) perfectly, even though this parent likely does not follow the code in such a way. One would not think an overly religious family would have the same dynamics as an alcoholic family, but years of teaching boundaries has shown the authors that the two types of families are similarly dysfunctional.

Attachment Templates and Theories

Very early childhood development may also play a critical role in one's ability to establish healthy physician-patient relationships. English psychiatrist John Bowlby and American psychologist Mary Ainsworth were primarily responsible for the attachment template child development theories[10]. Their combined work merged as they theorized that mother-child interaction was the key to the development of infants and young children. They theorized that a secure attachment to parents or

---

[10] Ainsworth MDS, Bowlby J. (1991). An ethological approach to personality development. *American Psychologist, 46*, 331–341.

caregivers before exploring the world on their own or facing unfamiliar or stressful situations is paramount to how children eventually behave as adults. They postulated that the relationship between the infant and mother (or primary caregiver) is responsible for shaping all future relationships and that a secure attachment allows children to focus, analyze their feelings, and recover from unexpected or traumatic events. They developed four attachment templates that over the years have been re-described and renamed, but the basic premise still exists:

Secure Attachment occurs when the mother or caregiver is nearby, accessible, responsive, and attentive to the infant. If the child perceives all these to be true, then the child feels loved, secure, and confident. Children who detect a secure attachment will have solid self-esteem and are more likely to explore their environment and be generally sociable. Thus, a secure attachment in infancy provides a platform for normal personality and social development as an adult.

Avoidant Attachment describes a parent who is unavailable or rejecting. The child thus decides that relying on others to meet their attachment needs is useless. They become self-centered, separate, and unresponsive to the needs of others.

Ambivalent Attachment is formed by an erratic and inconsistent parent. The parent may be intrusive at times and distant at others, and the child never knows what to expect. The child does not know how to interpret this inconsistency or intrusiveness, as they have no reliable or stable pattern to rely on. These children become anxious and fearful because they don't know what to expect from their caregiver. As they develop, they vacillate between availability and rejection. They argue but without resolution and have deep insecurities that can lead to over-attachment as an adult.

Disorganized Attachment is based on fear. Parents may be physically or verbally abusive. They are chaotic and random. This experience as a child later translates into an adult who either avoids relationships or can be extremely aggressive or abusive in relationships. Unfortunately, these children have been programmed to fail as adults.

As the child develops, attachments can form between a child and his or her siblings, other family members, teachers, and coaches, but it appears that the parents have the most influence on a child's ability to grow into a successful adult.

It's worth noting that you cannot erase your family background or attachments—they make you who you are; but, with self-awareness, education, and sometimes therapy, destructive coping mechanisms and behavior patterns can certainly be changed.

Hazan and Shaver (1990) developed a simple questionnaire to measure attachment patterns in adults. They based their survey on three categories instead of four: secure, avoidant, and anxious-resistant. They based their study results on the first 670 responses that were received after sending out 1,000 questionnaires. Fifty percent of respondents indicated they were secure, 30% avoidant, and 19% anxious-resistant.[11]

---

[11] Hazan C., Shaver, P. (1990).Romantic Love Conceptualized as an attachment process. *Journal of Personality and Social Psychology, 59,* 270–280.

Adults who are securely attached tend to have lasting, trusting, and long-term relationships. They enjoy a solid self-esteem and seek out social support and friends. They also have the ability to share their feelings with others. By contrast, the other attachment templates in one form or another tend to be socially inept, anxious, chaotic, distrustful, fearful, and generally lack all the aspects of emotional intelligence. Thus, according to the attachment template theory, 49% of those surveyed by Hazan and Shaver lacked at least some emotional intelligence, affecting their ability to form appropriate and healthy relationships in different aspects of their lives.

Many healthcare professionals would like to place themselves squarely in the "secure attachment template" category, in a family void of unhealthy roles and rules; or, perhaps, they admit to being outside these parameters but view themselves as having conquered the adversity they faced as children and teenagers. However, ignoring vast influences on your character and personality does a disservice to yourself and your patients, who give you the power to alter their physical and mental well-being.

If both your background and your patients' backgrounds are based on secure attachments, then the physician-patient relationship can probably have broader and somewhat more porous boundaries. On the other hand, more than 40% of us have attachment templates that are not secure. That signals a potential problem with many provider-patient relationships. In primary care and the mental health fields in particular, the relationship is more than casual, leaving room for more vague boundary lines. In these fields, and in most healthcare fields, evaluating your attachment template as well as those of your patients or clients may be necessary if you perceive a potential conflict or boundary issues. Of course, it may not always be possible to evaluate the patient's attachment template; a mental health professional can delve much further into a patient's background than a dermatologist, but being aware of where your patients are coming from can benefit your practice. Family roles and rules theory and attachment templates theory may also help you identify the patient or client that "drives you crazy" and why you continue to accept these patients even though they present a risk to you and your practice.

A provider who violates boundaries, feels uneasy about how to control boundaries, or is confused as to where those boundaries lie would do well not only to identify his or her family roles, rules, and attachment templates, but to be hypervigilant when scenarios arise that signal his or her boundaries are at risk of being violated or that he or she is about to violate the boundaries of the patient or client. I hope that by the conclusion of this book, you will have the knowledge and the tools to accomplish this.

We all want to believe that we are secure, intelligent, well-trained, and pretty much bullet-proof. Unfortunately, a false sense of security does not protect us from possibly committing boundary violations. There are professionals of many stripes that can assist a provider in overcoming the effects of a toxic family of origin and/or issues with poor infant attachments. While many of us might feel that course of action unnecessary, consider the influence roles, rules, and attachment templates might be having on the care you provide or your group practice.

Suggested Further Reading:
The Attachment Effect, Peter Lovenheim, Tarcher Perigee, 2018.

Family Systems and Life-Span Development, K Kreppner, Hillsdale, 1989.

"Patterns of Attachment: A Psychological Study of the Strange Situation," M Ainsworth, Psychology Press, 1978.

Chapter 3:
The Road to Boundary Violations

Although we might assume a provider is an educated professional immediately upon passing his or her exam, professional training does not end with formal education. It includes continual on-the-job learning and the consequences of mistakes, misjudgments, and just plain wrong guesses.

It is important to note that between the pressures to perform successfully and to do so cost-effectively, healthcare professionals in training take on a singular focus: do what needs to be done to get the degree. Thoughts about ethics and boundaries can become overshadowed by the realities of day-to-day healthcare practice. In this phase of career development, one learns from and reacts to experiences in ways that shape who they will become professionally and how they will behave in relationships with patients.

Training to be a healthcare professional requires a level of commitment, dedication, and effort that is more focused and intense than many other careers. Because providing healthcare is personal and involves vulnerability and trust, any practitioner-to-be is expected to embody a level of confidence and capability that separates him or her from the pack.

By the time medical training is complete, the candidate has endured sleep deprivation, amazing amounts work and study hours, and mounting stress from competition in the field. Throughout their training, medical professionals hear and come to believe that this demanding lifestyle is not only part of the process, but worth the end result—credentials and a well-respected career. However, one result of the pressure from years of training and accumulating knowledge can be an unhealthy tolerance for pressure and unreasonable expectations.

Akin to the toughening process athletes undertake in preparation for competition, medical training includes an emotional process that is designed to prepare a successful candidate for the continued demands of the profession. In the background of this training process buzzes the reality of the current healthcare climate. When anyone entrusts a loved one to the care of a healthcare provider at any level, they assume that their loved one is not only going to receive the best possible healthcare, but is also going to have the perfect outcome.

The expectation that all practitioners can provide perfect outcomes is woven into the hiring and staffing process of healthcare organizations. Hospitals and other healthcare organizations demand that every applicant has the highest qualifications and the best training possible to provide optimal outcomes in the specific job for which he or she is hired. The top leaders of every healthcare organization put pressure on their talent to provide exceptional quality of care regardless of career, purpose, perceived importance of the job, attained skill, or specialty training. Candidates often feel pressured to shorten the learning curve and out-perform any other candidate.

Another sign of "success" in medical training is the practitioner's ability to accomplish a task without asking for help. In many areas of medicine, students are often told directly that, beyond a certain point, asking for help is a sign of weakness. (Clearly, this is a destructive message, though a relatively common one in healthcare.)

These rigorous expectations begin as soon as an individual submits an application to medical school and continues all the way to retirement.

Success, Power, and Distance

What, if any, logical reasoning would establish such a pressurized, process? First, let's look at the root of success and leadership. Whether a provider aspires to be a strong team player in the center of a chain of providers, such as a team leader in home health care; a director of a department; or a solo provider of a singular service (such as a therapist), success as a provider involves an exchange of power. Here are some examples:

- An athlete reclines on the physical therapy table to allow a physical therapist to begin moving an injured joint in an effort to restore range of motion and extend pain tolerance. The athlete must relinquish power to and trust the physical therapist during this interaction.
- An elderly patient in a skilled nursing facility with a healing total hip replacement requires assistance with bathing and must allow herself to be physically and emotionally vulnerable in the process.
- A veteran with post-traumatic stress disorder sits with an individual therapist and agrees to relive the nightmares and intrusive thoughts that interfere with his life and send him on an emotional rollercoaster. He shares these thoughts believing that the therapist has tools and information that will change the daily pain he faces.

- A director of nursing views the census and sees that the overall patient load is 20% bigger than usual, and that more than half the patients are considered serious. The usual staffing plan assumes that 35–40% of patients are in serious condition. On top of that, the lead charge nurse is out on medical leave. As he makes rounds, he asks each staff member to verify that the needs of the patients are being met, relying on the honest answers and trust he has placed in them to ensure the best possible patient care for the shift.

In each of these situations, the patient relinquishes power and transfers trust to the provider. In turn, the provider must create some emotional distance between him- or herself and the patient. This is where the power equation becomes unbalanced. Although some distance is necessary to help the professional be objective and see the whole picture, too much distance can be detrimental to a patient-provider relationship. For example, a certain emotional distance provides objectivity when a patient or client is in pain, but excessive emotional distance may make the provider numb to the patient's pain experience. It is therefore helpful to think of "distance" on a spectrum with "too distant" at one end and "enmeshed" at the other.

Not only is there a degree of distance between the provider and his or her patients, but there is also distance between the individuals in charge of a healthcare organization and the people the organization cares for. The CEO may care deeply for patients and may truly want to provide optimal care, but he or she must make decisions for the organization based on performance statistics, profits, state and federal regulations, etc., not on how Mrs. Smith in room 7 is feeling after her surgery today. In healthcare, often the individual with the greatest power is the most distant from the patient.

Regardless of where the power lies, the weight of consequence ends up on the patient or whomever is at the lowest end of the power differential. This is a bit easier to understand in the corporate world of workers, managers, supervisors, executives, etc. However, the same inverse pyramid applies to educators seeking tenure, small business owners trying to survive, clergy trying to salvage a struggling church, etc. The key issue is the power differential that comes from the responsibility and trust that is exchanged in any type of business relationship. This kind of responsibility defines a fiduciary relationship, where one person places complete confidence in another, mainly because he or she believes that person has superior knowledge and training.

In healthcare, business, education, and other high-stakes fields, a leader's decision might have a significant effect on the wellbeing, emotional state, and financial stability of an individual's personal life. But in healthcare specifically, how an organization handles its fiduciary responsibility can sometimes mean life or death.

The Consequences of Medical Training and Career Development

Training to accept a fiduciary responsibility that ultimately affects patients' health and wellbeing is intense and can, through its necessary demands, become insensitive and emotionless. Common sense might imply that in teaching an individual to provide care, one would want to also teach compassion. Oddly enough, this is the very paradox of the training process and has not been addressed until recently. In the process of developing successful healthcare professionals, institutions now see the need for a process that acknowledges its intensity and provides a mechanism to help the professional better cope with it. Individuals without the constitutional capacity to endure the ongoing stresses of medical training, professional responsibility, and general life stress in these careers could suffer in a system that ignores the inherent pressures. Much of this pressure and intensity are related to not only the responsibility, but also the vulnerability inherent in such power differentials.

Elements of the Provider-Patient Relationship

Both the patient and the practitioner bring something to the relationship. Often, a patient enters a provider's care feeling vulnerable. He or she feels a sense of need, urgency, incompetence, and dependence. If a patient cannot entrust his or her wellbeing—or even his or her life—to the professional, he or she is stuck feeling helpless. In addition, the *professional* brings things to the relationship that enhance trust and ease the transfer of power. These include the tools of the trade; procedural knowledge; the ability to project relief of pain, tension, or stress; awareness of potential outcomes; and autonomy. (As a cautionary note, the professional who has been repeatedly successful in the past may feel infallible and become over-confident.)

The following are what the patient brings to the provider-patient relationship, thus contributing to the inherently stressful power differential:

Vulnerability

For any human to transfer the power of fiduciary responsibility to a professional, the recipient of care feels vulnerable. That vulnerability may come from physical illness, financial instability, the need for nursing care, or from receiving physical or emotional therapy. Remember, the individual's sense of overall wellbeing hangs in the balance, even when the provider is not at risk of causing physical harm. By the time a person has made the appointment with the provider, the sense of despair, regardless of how superficial or deep, has highlighted the sense of need, fear, and confusion that fuels vulnerability.

Need

Vulnerability is rooted in a sense of need. Most people rarely make a spur-of-the-moment decision to ask for help from a professional. Out of a sense of vulnerability comes the rational solution-seeking process that leads a patient to think, "I need help." The desire to fix this threat or deficit heightens the sense of need, which leads the individual to contact the professional.

Example: A 76-year-old widow has been limping on a painful hip for some time, and her doctor has referred her for physical therapy. She is in pain, alone, and is terrified of being hurt. In addition, she is still grieving the loss of her husband of 52 years and is anxious about disrobing and allowing a male physician to move her leg and hip. She is vulnerable physically and emotionally.

Urgency

At the intersection of vulnerability and need is a sense of urgency that can drive a person to seek the assistance of a professional. Urgency comes from a deep sense of doom, pain, or fear, whether it is based in reality or fantasy. The problem with urgency is that it is defined by the urgent person. What feels urgent to one person may not feel urgent to another. If a patient has seen a vaguely similar situation or symptoms in someone they know, and that individual had a catastrophic result, the sense of urgency mounts. In many cases, no amount of reassurance will lessen the sense of urgency. However, the power the patient has assigned to a medical professional can help him or her enter the relationship with trust and a sense of safety in the storm of urgency.

Example: The widow in the previous example may have had a friend or family member who ignored pain in the hip and had metastatic cancer to that bone, heralding a rapid course to death. She is not exaggerating her fear, but is, in reality, acting from real experience. Her ability to trust her diagnosing physician and the providers to whom she is referred will be key to decreasing her sense of urgency.

Incompetence

When patients reach the point of asking a healthcare professional for help, they have run out of options, made all their best guesses, and searched the internet for all the worst-case scenarios. All their best research and efforts have failed to lessen their fears and reduce the sense of urgency, leaving them feeling incompetent to take care of the problem. With the stage set by vulnerability and urgency, the next step is an internal declaration of incompetence. Placing one's self in the hands of another with the urgent sense of incompetence crystallizes the fiduciary relationship.

Dependence

By nature of their medical training and licensure, patients often assume that healthcare providers have the answers on which one can rely. Thus, begins a relationship in which patients depend on providers for those answers. The handshake, whether physical or emotional, that christens the relationship represents a tacit, often insoluble agreement to this dependence. A few examples of the type of dependence that can exist between professional and patient include:

- *Financial*
    Whoever pays for healthcare fosters financial dependence. This is an unavoidable reality. Healthcare choices are limited when patients have to choose an in-network co-pay, higher out-of-network co-pay, or must pay the full fee for services. Even with insurance, the patient always has to gamble whether insurance will pay or reimburse them. A harsh reality for healthcare providers is that a percentage of our insured patients are not seeing their first choice in care when they see us.

Example: Many very specialized practitioners and centers have elected not to participate in some health insurance plans, including Medicare. An athlete with a torn ligament in her knee may really want to go to the surgeon who has successfully treated numerous team members. However, that surgeon no longer accepts her insurance plan. Therefore, she is seeing her second or third choice. Can she trust this new surgeon as much as she could her first choice?

- *Social*

Many social factors contribute to the choices one makes regarding healthcare services. Often, social circles are a huge source of stories about providers and the care they provide. In fact, these stories are absolutely true for each individual, whether or not they represent the reality of the whole. Sometimes, not choosing a popular physician, facility, or route of care can lead friends and peers to reject, criticize, or have negative expectations for the individual seeking care. In this way, the needs patients have for healthcare can fall counter to their social ties and lead them to feel ostracized. Friends and family can offer messages of approval or disapproval about healthcare. When friends and family send a message that the patient's choice of treatment or provider is favorable in their eyes, the patient's chance of adhering to treatment and, therefore, having a better outcome, dramatically increases. Here are some examples:

Example: John has been a member of the Rotary Club for many years. Everyone he knows who has received physical therapy has seen Dr. Z. Unfortunately, John's insurance doesn't work with Dr. Z, so John is seeing Dr. K. His longstanding sense of defiance and "I'll show them" attitude has encouraged him to show his peers that his plan of care (and physician) is just as good as theirs. John is therefore extremely diligent and precise in following his physical therapist's suggestions. In this way, the sense that he was *not* doing what everybody approved of led him to a better, positive outcome.

Example: Deborah has always been fascinated with being on the fringe. Most of her friends are very active in holistic healing and avoid seeing traditional healthcare providers. She has tried acupuncture, herbal remedies, and many non-traditional means to reduce the pain in her back. Her decision to go to a physician and receive physical therapy in a typical, traditional health system has led to many cynical messages from her friends about this decision. She enters her therapy with many questions and doubts, many of which have come from her long-held beliefs about non-traditional medicine. Her tenacity and diligence in her treatment will depend heavily on her provider's ability to gain her trust.

Example: Marge's husband had a dramatic adverse response to medical treatment, possibly mislabeled as an allergic reaction to a specific antibiotic. When her sister was placed on that particular antibiotic, Marge demanded that her sister call the physician and refuse to take it, reiterating the horror story of her husband's experience.

As we can see, social messages can both help and hinder a patient's decision regarding whether and where to seek help. Strongly held beliefs about how diet, exercise, or other preventative measures might reduce the problem can add to the resistance to seek help, fuel denial about the seriousness of the problem, and delay crucial decisions.

Friends, family, and providers can also put pressure on their loved ones to be "good patients." The messages we carry from our families of origin, cultural backgrounds, and life experiences weigh heavily on how easily patients give their trust to a provider, deeply affecting how they respond to and receive care.

- *Intellectual*

    Each provider's communication style is unique to our task, our field, and our education and training. In our language, complex words and terms can communicate large amounts of information to another provider.

    To a physician or nurse, "Let's get a CBC and see what your white count is," translates into "I want to do a blood test to see if you have an infection, find out if it is bacterial or viral, and understand the extent of the infection." The latter is understandable to the layperson, while the former might not be. The dependence on us to translate, and translate well, will affect patients' intellectual dependence on providers. This can put us in double jeopardy; if we translate too well, we may terrify the patient needlessly, but, if done poorly, we may reinforce the patient's sense of incompetence and ignorance.

Other Factors Contributing to the Power Differential

    The knowledge healthcare professionals work so hard to attain and what it represents creates a strong power differential. Our patients generally lack this knowledge—they don't know what their stomach pain might mean, or how to treat it, or the chances that treatment will be successful or what their response to treatment means. Even though physicians put on their pants one leg at a time like everyone else, some patients regard physicians' knowledge as infallible. Patients often don't see practitioners grasp for answers, research symptoms, and ask colleagues for opinions regarding diagnoses; rather, they may consider this knowledge natural intelligence.

Next to physicians' knowledge, the tools, access, and power provided by licensure can widen the gap between provider and patient. We can run the ECG machine, use ultrasound to enhance physical therapy, or take an X-ray. Physicians can do something as simple as getting the patient an extra blanket or as complex as removing a tumor wrapped around an organ. We have access to and an understanding of these tools that extends far beyond that of the patient.

Power to Prescribe/Direct Treatment

The power to prescribe and direct treatment—a power granted to us by licensure—is a clear power differential. Even if a patient is well educated and has information as to which medication he or she might most benefit from, the patient still cannot attain it without a licensed healthcare professional with the legal capacity to prescribe it. Additionally, patients know the power of medication—albeit, sometimes incorrectly. One only has to reflect on the number of times a primary care provider has to say, "This is clearly a viral infection and antibiotics won't help it go away any quicker," to grasp the magic that prescribed medication can instill in a patient. Likewise, our legal power and ability to perform procedures on a patient's body is another clear-cut power differential. Whether it is a tumor, a muscle in spasm, a soiled bed linen, or an IV the patient wants out, the procedural skills a provider has are another factor in widening the power gap between patient and provider.

As healthcare providers, we are also wise to remind ourselves that not everyone remains calm around blood, much less can find the wherewithal to cut into the human body. The skill to take charge of one's own emotions within the power differential and to not only take action, but take charge of the needs of another, requires tapping into many levels of the knowledge and experience of our training. These qualities give us power in the eyes of our patients that adds to our overall influence on the patient.

Power to Select Treatments

Our pharmaceutical and therapeutic "pantry" is among the greatest source of power we have. If we are honest with ourselves, it is the medication and therapy that cure the patient, not the provider.

Another source of power is a provider's autonomy to choose *how* to present medication. The style in which a provider presents a plan of care can influence the patient's willingness to comply and belief that it will work, thus affecting patient outcomes.[12, 13] In addition, much of what a provider says and how he or she says it can have a significant effect on the patient's mood and outlook regarding the illness.

Example: A caring assistant in the recovery room may provide a patient with a warm blanket, a smile, and reassurance that "This will help you be more comfortable." The care team then finds that the patient voices less acute pain. On the other hand, a busy staff

---

[12] Holden, C. (2002). Neuroscience, Drugs and Placebos Look Alike in the Brain. *Science, 295*, 947

[13] Petrovic P, et al. (2002). Placebo and Opioid Analgesia-Imaging and Shared Neural Network. *Science, 295*, 1737–1740.

member may loosely toss the same warmed blanket over a patient with the remark, "Here, this should help," and scurry away, only to be called back repeatedly to address the patient's complaints about pain.

Power of Knowing Potential Outcomes

Practitioners hold the power of seeing into the future—no, not really, but we do have the ability to predict a reasonable outcome and treatment response. How a practitioner communicates what a treatment response looks like will affect the patient's outcome.

Example: Dr. M.'s nurse, Vicki, routinely tells his worried parents of pediatric patients that a child may continue to have fever for 48 to 72 hours after the first dose of an antibiotic. This is likely to increase the parents' attention to treating the fever, rather than focusing on whether the medication is working. Dr. P.'s nurse, Loretta, does not provide worried parents with the same information and complains in the doctor's lounge about how parents are "always" calling at midnight on the first day of antibiotics because the child's fever persists.

Power of Communication

A provider's communication style can enhance or inhibit the provider-patient relationship. For example, speaking in a loud, demanding tone of voice can greatly upset a patient; being curt or blunt can be devastating; and not providing clear directions can leave a patient bewildered.

One of the most intensely powerful forms of communication is the lack of it. Silence, omission, or inattention to detail can be a dangerous source of power for the healthcare provider.

Example: A patient is about to undergo treatment for a painful ankle and asks, "Is this going to hurt?" Whether the provider says, "Humph," "Not at all," "Probably," or "It may, just let me know if it's too uncomfortable," can dramatically affect the treatment outcome.

The importance, rationality, or silliness of the question to the provider is totally irrelevant. What matters is how important that question is to the patient, and how it is answered could potentially affect the patient's state of mind and outlook for the day, or until the next visit, or for much longer.

Power of Style

Professor Albert Mehrabian published an article on communication in 1967[14] and, while somewhat inaccurately interpreted by many, it has been used to describe the degree to which words affect communication. The important message that came out of this work was that *how* we say things is as important as what we say and that both are dramatically affected by how we look, especially our facial expressions. For example, if a patient has asked a question that, to the provider, seems like an unnecessary question, and that provider smiles and pats the

---

[14] Mehrabian, A., and Ferris, S.R. (1967). Inference of Attitudes from Nonverbal Communication in Two Channels, *Journal of Consulting Psychology, 31*, 48–258

patient's hands then exits the room, then the patient might interpret these communication signals as dismissing or patronizing.

Example: A neurosurgeon is well known in emergency rooms for his compassion after he attended a fatally injured teenager in the ER. When it was obvious that the injuries were lethal, he called for the parents. When they walked into the room, he stood at the bedside holding the young patient's hand with tears running down his cheeks. Not a word was said until one of the parents asked him, "Can we turn off the machines and let her go?" Volumes of compassion, care, and information were exchanged without words.

Power of Information

Finally, one of the most difficult areas to navigate as a healthcare provider is what information to give a patient and when:

- Should a patient be informed about a cancer diagnosis in the recovery room?
- Who shares the chances of a negative outcome and when?
- Does an aide give a family information about a comatose patient?

Anyone who has had a lump examined may recall that the threat of a cancer diagnosis hung in the room, in the minds of the patient and the provider. Balancing the importance of diagnosis and treatment with the emotional impact of that information is a part of the art of healthcare. While a concerned professional does not want to panic a patient with the worst-case scenario all the time, to omit a genuine concern because communicating it is uncomfortable can risk overwhelming a patient later. In reality, much trial-and-error will go into learning how to explain to a patient that a lump may likely be a fatty tumor, but that a cancer of some sort is always a possibility. To erroneously present the patient with a cancer diagnosis with what turns out to be a soft-tissue tumor precipitates a patient's needless worry, fear, and questioning. On the other end of the spectrum, a patient is likely to feel blindsided by a negative result because the provider did not communicate the possibility of cancer in an attempt to avoid undue stress and worry.

Keeping in mind that the patient's primary concern will be their worst-case fear, the provider is wise to rely on all the information possible before giving a final answer. Patients are likely to be overwhelmed by specific percentages and statistics that mean much to the clinician and very little to the layperson. Giving general information with plenty of room (and time and availability) to ask questions is the foundation of trust in this process. An essential and useful question to end this process is a simple: "What do *you* worry about the most?" Simply hearing the question and having the concern validated without dismissal may allay far more fears than statistics. Finally, when in doubt, seek wisdom from another trusted and experienced provider.

Power of Analgesia (Pain Relief)

When treating a medical condition, whether by intervening or maintaining comfort, the provider has the potential power to alleviate pain. After all, the ultimate goal of any healthcare process is relieving the patient's distress, pain, and fear. Any noticeable reduction in the negative aspects of an illness gives the patient hope and magnifies the somewhat magical influence that the provider has in healing. Even if that feeling doesn't last, it leaves a lasting impression about how a patient feels toward that provider in the future. A patient who has a positive result when placing trust in a provider is likely to seek out that provider the next time he or she has a need and might generally trust all providers a bit more.

Power of Experience

Another often-overlooked source of power is our experience. As providers, we have usually *seen* the results of whatever treatment or guidance we are providing. A patient who has sought out our care, even the most routine care, may have a bit of knowledge about how the issue is supposed to resolve. However, it can still be difficult for the patient to navigate through fear and vulnerability well enough to believe that he or she is going to get better, recover fully, or find relief from pain without actually seeing results with his or her own eyes.

As healthcare providers, it's important to understand how emotions work, and have a good level of emotional intelligence. For example, keep in mind that many people who feel negative emotions (such as those that often arise in a time of illness) believe they will always feel that way—psychology terms this "affective forecasting" or predicting how one is going to feel in the future based on how they feel now. People are also apt to thinking that their negative emotions accurately reflect real life (psychologists call this emotional reasoning).

Example: An 82-year-old woman goes into the hospital sensing dread and doom because she is acutely aware of her age. She assumes she will die in the hospital, even if she came in for a highly treatable and curable condition. Of course, being elderly presents risk, but the patient, believing her sense of doom, believes with near certainty that she will never leave that hospital. The attending physician gives her a glimpse of hope by reassuring her that he has provided this treatment before and has seen it work. He offers her concrete and real-life examples about past experiences of patients like her, which positively influence her frame of mind.

Power of Autonomy

A subtle part of the power differential between healthcare providers and patients is the reality that, when we leave the exam room, the patient takes 100% of the problem home with them and we do not. The patient may not have any measurable relief from the pain, fear, or need that brought them into the exam room (and indeed, might not be able to resume their normal lives). This is another example of how patients are aware that they depend heavily on us, much more than we depend on them. Even if a provider's emotions rise and fall with each patient he or she sees, the provider does not always express it. In fact, we are trained to contain and even suppress these experiences so that they stay ours and do not affect the patient. Although hiding or expressing emotions can serve providers well in some instances, patients who are feeling vulnerable may feel that the provider is unflappable, highlighting their own feelings of weakness.

Power of Perceived Infallibility

As wise healthcare providers, we know that we have made and will make mistakes. However, when a provider has received the trust of a patient and has simply done a good job providing prompt, positive care, the patient may place the provider on the pedestal of infallibility. Whether this impression is deserved or the provider participated in getting on that pedestal, it may be the way the patient compensates for his or her own sense of vulnerability and many other aspects of humanness. (It's much more comforting to think that your doctor never makes mistakes than thinking of him or her as just another human, just as apt at making a mistake as the rest of us.) One sure way for a provider to eventually damage a patient's trust is to abandon all humility and egotistically agree with the idea that he or she is infallible. Eventually, the patient is going to realize that healthcare providers are human, and consciously or unconsciously, they will be forced to take us off that pedestal.

The more power patients perceive us to have, the stronger their own sense of ignorance and helplessness. The patient may fear losing the provider and have less incentive to question the provider's plans, recommendations, or directions. In addition, only one *perceived* harsh or negative response from a provider regarding a question or challenge to the treatment may lead the patient to become unwilling to challenge or ask questions.

[Chart] The Language of Power Differentials

Patient	Provider
I feel sick. I don't know what is wrong. I don't know if I can afford treatment. I can't afford the medication. I believe you can make me well. My life is in your hands. Nobody else can do what you do. Nobody could do what you DID.	I'm the [doctor, nurse, therapist, etc.] here. I can help you. I have the training. I have samples. You can trust me. I'll work with your insurance. This is part of my examination.[15] Nobody else has the [technique, skills, or knowledge] that I have. I've known you the longest. I know your whole family.

Power of Objectivity

Part and parcel of training to be a professional is the necessary distance we call "objectivity." We must learn to be with a patient in pain or in crisis and remain calm in order to identify and provide the necessary treatment. If we are overwhelmed or taken in by the patient's experience, we begin to cloud the treatment with our own feelings and may give the patient more or less than they need, or, in a less useful scenario, give them what *we* need and not necessarily what *they* need. A

---

[15] Variations of this statement are one of the common recollections reported when patient has been the victim of a sexual boundary violation.

63

strong and professional measure of objectivity is essential to being a good healthcare provider. However, if we believe that our view of the patient is an impenetrable one-way mirror and we are never influenced by the physician-patient relationship, we are accepting an illusion. The illusion becomes like "night vision" or "blue vision" glasses that filter out intense blue light and improve vision. After a short while, our brains adjust to this altered vision and can identify a spectrum of colors as we know them, such as traffic lights. We begin to believe that we have accurate color perception with these lenses on. However, you wouldn't want to choose a color with which to paint your house with such glasses on. Likewise, the belief that we are 100% objective and have no bias in any professional decision is risky.

In the midst of developing our professional demeanor, we present ourselves to the world as confident, calm, and collected. Patients put their trust in us whether this is the second time we have treated their problem or the second thousandth time. The provider has a fiduciary responsibility to care for the patient in the best way possible.

Most of us can recall the first time we performed fully in the role as a practitioner. Our job was to take charge, handle it, and make the patient feel better. We accomplish this despite our possible insecurity, fear, and confusion. With practice and further demands from education and training, the provider is expected to be therapeutically neutral in all situations. Therefore, the provider must defer or suppress any negative reactions or emotions, as well as some of the more positive aspects of the situation. The greatest threat to the patient-provider relationship is a provider who begins to believe he or she has no fear or uncertainty, perhaps becoming defensive about being questioned. To be unwilling to be mistaken risks patient lives and ignores potential alternatives that may affect the patient's outcome.

An unfortunate side effect of developing a hard shell of objectivity is that providers are often encouraged, both overtly and covertly, to deny their own sadness, fear, anxiety, and grief. Providers are often treated and treat themselves as if they are not part of the patient experience.

For example, when a certain procedure, diagnosis, or treatment with a past patient happens to be associated, in our minds, with the most dramatic outcome, positive or negative, the memories of that patient are automatically associated with mental pictures, sounds, smells and a myriad of other sensory experiences. Other physical or visceral feelings may present themselves unconsciously along with the memory. As we become objective in any situation, we suppress the conscious and sensory components of a memory and may only have a deep "inner" sense of the situation. While it may seem easier to push the memories and its associated feelings from our focus, they affect us nonetheless. Memories of a patient who deeply impacted us may begin to drive clinical decision-making without us knowing it. Healthcare providers must understand and recognize that *every patient and every procedure* represents a pixel in the decision-making picture. This includes the shadows of loss, frustration, and anger related to certain patients, as well as positive aspects of patient encounters. Accordingly, every patient who dies, whether of natural causes or the direct or indirect result of treatment, is a loss. One residual effect of these inevitable losses can be the ever-nagging question of whether the provider observed the loss or was a part of creating the loss. While a patient's death is rarely the result of a single act by a single provider, the provider will still question him- or herself. The lessons learned from mistakes hone the provider into a better and more accurate practitioner but can also leave an indelible mark on the ego. It's wise to create a boundary between memory of a past experience and the current situation at hand; or, at the very least, acknowledge that some emotions can threaten your usual patient boundaries.

These factors are crucial components in building healthy boundaries and avoiding boundary violations. As providers, we must understand the power of the trust that our patients place in us, including how that trust can be both positive and negative. In addition, we must understand all our points of vulnerability, not only to prevent them from causing the patient negative feelings, but also to ensure they do not cause boundary violations.

Being aware of your own vulnerabilities might include seemingly simple situations, such as the following:

- A patient reminds me too much of a mean Grade 2 teacher. I need to be very aware of my level of patience with her and ensure that I am responding to the patient and not to my residual anger and hurt from that teacher.
- Communicating with patients with difficult or just different speaking accents from mine can be frustrating. Speaking more loudly at them

does not help them communicate better with me.

- Patients with medical problems or physical limitations that remind us of family members may dampen our enthusiasm in the unconscious interest of avoiding the pain we witnessed in a loved one, thus giving our patients less optimal care.

Each of these scenarios shows the beginnings of flaws in our internal boundaries that become openings for greater boundary violations if we don't take care. We are all wise to ask ourselves what is at play any time we are providing more than just routine care.

Reminder: The provider is at the top of the power differential and is, by standard, always responsible for the maintenance of boundaries in the professional relationship.

Because so many factors are at play in any interaction with a patient, the skillful provider must enter the relationship with objectivity and an open mind, while acknowledging that his or her own biases and vulnerabilities are always present. While past professional experiences can affect the care a practitioner provides, so can personal experiences, and this must be recognized as well. For example, I recall one session with the 72-year-old patient I was seeing for therapy who wore the same perfume that my mother usually wore. I specifically noticed this within a month of my mother's death. Though the patient did not report anything unusual about the session, I am quite certain that I was distracted and less than 100% efficacious in that session. This kind of subtle, mostly unconscious distraction can weaken our boundaries and open the door for the minor transgressions that allow deeper violations to occur if the provider does not face them openly and consciously.

The decision to provide healthcare to others is one that is built on the foundation of all our experiences in life. Our work and our successes continue to shape our daily practice. Being aware of these factors is crucial to avoiding boundary violations. Understanding what makes a provider so powerful in the eyes of the patient can help you adjust your relationship with patients appropriately. Also understanding and being mindful about how past experience and memories might affect your care is another step toward knowing yourself, the unique patient-provider bond, and where to set up your boundaries.

Take-Aways
- Earning a medical degree or any other professional degree does not make you "educated."
- The healthcare provider is always at the top of the power differential and is always responsible for maintaining proper boundaries.
- Understanding your own vulnerabilities can help you create healthy relationships with patients.

Chapter 4:
The Influence of Empathy

Empathy is a necessary, meaningful, and critical skill to the delivery of compassionate healthcare. However, it is a double-edged sword: too much is a potential problem for the caregiver, too little is a potential problem for the patient. A caregiver's empathy can be a gift, but as in most things, an overabundance can be a substantial risk and a burden. The overly empathetic individual many times is without boundaries, even to the point of codependency. Conversely, the narcissistic provider who lacks empathy can be an ineffective provider and possibly harm the patient. Neither extremes are helpful in the therapeutic relationship; in fact, they pose a risk to everyone involved. This chapter explains empathy and its relationship to boundaries. More importantly, we discuss how to use empathy to enhance care.

The Importance and Benefits of Empathy

The importance of empathy probably needs no explanation, but providers must recognize that our reputations as healers depend on our ability to be empathetic. Dr. Helen Reiss, the director of the Empathy and Relational Science Program and associate professor of psychiatry at Harvard Medical School, summarizes literature on the topic to these points:

- Medical professionals who communicate with empathy have higher patient satisfaction ratings.[16]

---

[16] H Reiss, 2012, Why Empathy, http://empathetics.com/why-empathy

- More than 80% of malpractice claims are the result of communication failures, and the likelihood of an unhappy outcome is correlated to low physician empathy.[17, 18]
- Patients who experience empathetic care have better medical outcomes.[19, 20, 21]
- Adherence to treatment recommendations increases when medical professionals deliver patient-centered, compassionate care.[22]
- Communicating empathetically increases clinician job satisfaction and reduces burnout.[23, 24, 25]
- Enhanced empathetic care and physician well-being are highly correlated.[26]
- Empathetic clinician communication improves the quality of interactions with others, including patients, their families, colleagues, and loved ones. [27]

Empathy is what distinguishes us from computers practicing medicine. The good news is that empathy and

---

[17] Hickson,GB,Federspiel CF, Pichert JW, JAMA, 2002, 2951-2957

[18] Levinson W, Roter D, Mullolly J, JAMA, 1997,553-559

[19] Hojat M, Louis DZ, Markham FW, Acad Med, 2011, 359-364

[20] Rakel DP, Family Med, 2009, 494-501

[21] Kaptchuk TJ, Conboy LA, Kelly JM, BMJ, 2008, 999-1003

[22] Halpern J, J Gen Internal Med, 2007,696-700

[23] Krasner MS, JAMA, 2009, 1284-1293

[24] Shanafelt T, JAMA, 2009, 1338-1340

[25] West C, JAMA, 2011,952-960

[26] Shanafelt T, J Gen Internal Med, 2005, 559-564

[27] Halpern J, Med, Health Care Philosophy, 2014, 301-311

empathetic communication are learnable skills that can be taught both in the classroom and by mentoring.

Acceptance and Evolution of Empathy in Healthcare

A discussion of empathy must involve how we view ourselves, and more importantly, how we view others. George Bernard Shaw may have said it best in his play *Pygmalion*, "The great secret, Eliza, is not having bad manners or good manners, but having the same manner for all human souls. In short, behaving as if you were in heaven, where there are no third-class carriages, and one soul is as good as another."

NJ Rohrhoft, a senior medical student, clearly understood the role empathy plays in care when he wrote in a 2012 issue of the *New England Journal of Medicine*, "The caring of patients should begin with caring *about* them. We must not forget to ask 'how things are going.' It is the central challenge of our time as medicine evolves."[28] Empathy, as it was first described by EB Titchener, an Australian psychologist, meant mimicking another's feelings. His theory was that empathy evolved from one imitating the distress of another. Sympathy, on the other hand, is acknowledging the distress of another without actually sharing what the other person is feeling.

Empathy in the clinical setting has evolved as medicine has evolved. Sir William Osler in 1912 said, "Physicians should neutralize their emotions to the point that they feel nothing in response to suffering." In 1964, Herrman Blumgart, a noted professor of medicine and medical historian at the Harvard

---

[28] Rohrhoft, NJ. (2012). What Life is Like. *New Eng Journal of Medicine*,366:8.

Medical School stated in the *New England Journal of Medicine*: "Neutral empathy involves carefully observing a patient to predict his responses to illness. The neutrally empathetic physician will do what needs to be done without feeling grief, regret, or other difficult emotions." This approach, which required physicians to ignore or put aside empathy, was more than likely harmful to all involved, but was an attitude many physicians adopted.

Empathy Defined

Empathy has been defined in many ways by many authors, and it is often used interchangeably with sympathy; there is no universal agreement on what either means. In general, empathy is defined as the ability to identify with or understand another's situation or feelings (key word is "feelings") by putting yourself in someone else's shoes. Sympathy on the other hand is less personal and is defined as a feeling of pity or sorrow for the distress of another.

The essence of an empathetic person is the innate or learned ability to step out of your experience and into another person's. To do this, one must recognize it, feel it, understand it, and relay it to the other person. The experience can be physical, mental, emotional, intellectual, spiritual, or all of the above. Empathy arouses compassion in most of us, allowing us to connect and care about others. It is a critical attribute or skill for making good relationships, whether they are with patients, patients' families, friends, spouses, children, parents, partners, or co-workers. Everyone benefits from your empathy. It is based in part on the skill of active listening and not being distracted by your own parallel emotions, prejudices, or pre-conceived evaluations of the patient or their presentation in your treatment room.

The Neuroscience of Empathy

For many years, empathy was thought to be a personality trait, similar to good bedside manner. You either had it or you didn't. Behavioral and neuroscience disciplines now agree that it not only has a physiological basis mediated by the brain, but it can (and should) be taught and modeled. Jean Decety and Philip Jackson wrote in 2006:

> *There is strong evidence that, in the domain of emotion processing and empathetic understanding, people use the same neural circuits for themselves and for others. These circuits provide for a functional bridge between the first-person and third-person information, which paves the way for intersubjective transactions between self and others. These circuits can also be activated when one adopts the perspective of the other. However, were this bridging between self and other absolute, experiencing another's distress state as one's own experience could lead to empathetic over-arousal, in which the focus would then become one's own feelings of stress rather than the other's need. Self-agency and emotion-regulatory mechanisms thus play a crucial role in maintaining a boundary between self and other.*

The authors went on to state that based on functional MRI research, the insula—the lobe in the center of the cerebral hemisphere that is situated deeply between the lips of the sylvian fissure—is involved in monitoring the physiological state of the body. It receives direct input from the body's major pain pathway. Interestingly, both the anterior cingulate cortex and the insula are found to be activated by the mere sight of pain in others.[29]

A study published in *The Journal of Neuroscience* in 2013 enhances the previous research by identifying that the tendency to be egocentric is innate for human beings, but that a part of your brain recognizes this fact and corrects itself. This occurs in the right supramarginal gyrus. The right supramarginal gyrus of the brain is the junction that connects the thinking, feeling, and action portions of the brain. When it is disrupted, it is difficult to exhibit empathy. For example, the brain is much less apt to correct this lack of empathy when it does not function properly or when we have to make particularly quick decisions. When given the chance, the right supramarginal gyrus helps us distinguish our own emotional state from that of others and is responsible for our empathy and compassion. This area of the brain is part of the cerebral cortex and approximates the parietal, temporal, and frontal lobes. Tania Singer, the principal investigator of the study, stated:

When assessing the world around us and our fellow humans, we use ourselves as a yardstick and tend to project our own emotional state onto others. While cognition research has already studied this phenomenon in detail, nothing is known about how it works on an emotional level. It was assumed that

---

[29] Decety, J., Jackson, P. (2006). A Social Neuroscience Perspective on Empathy. *Current Directions in Psychological Science, 15*, 54–58.

our own emotional state can distort our understanding of other people's emotions, in particular if these are completely different to our own. But this emotional egocentricity had not been measured before.

The right supramarginal gyrus ensures that we can decouple our perception of ourselves from others. When the neurons in this part of the brain were disrupted in the course of the research, the participants found it difficult to stop projecting their own feelings and circumstances onto others. Quick decisions also disrupted their accuracy.

Researchers concluded that when we are in a comfortable and agreeable situation, it is more difficult to empathize with another person's suffering. The participants' own emotions distorted their assessment of the other people's feelings. The participants who were feeling good themselves assessed their partners' negative experiences as less severe than they actually were. In contrast, those who had just had an unpleasant experience assessed their partners' good experience less positively.[30]

Along the same line as this research, an article published in 2014 in the *Journal of Psychiatric Research* by Stefan Ropke found that individuals who suffer from narcissistic personality disorder have less gray matter in the left anterior insula of the cerebral cortex. Their conclusion, which is not yet proven, is that narcissistic traits are the result of structural abnormalities of the brain. The researchers found that the degree to which a person was able to exhibit empathy was tied to the volume of

---

[30] Bergland, Chris. (2013). The Athletes Way [blog].

gray matter in this area of the brain, both in the group of healthy individuals and among those with narcissistic personality disorder. The finding suggested that regardless of personality type, the left anterior insula plays an important role in feeling and compassion.[31]

Research conducted by the Department of Psychology of the University of Chicago and published in *Frontiers in Human Neuroscience* in 2013 found the neurobiological roots of psychopathic behavior—which is partly defined by a lack of empathy. Researchers wrote:

When highly psychopathic participants imagined pain to themselves, they showed a typical neural response within the anterior insula, anterior midcingulate cortex, somatosensory cortex, and the right amygdala. The research suggested the increase in brain activity in these regions was unusually pronounced, suggesting that psychopaths are sensitive to the thought of pain but are unable to put themselves in someone else's shoes and feel that pain. When participants imagined pain to others, these regions failed to become active in highly psychopathic individuals. In a sadistic twist, when imagining others in pain, psychopaths actually showed an increased response in the ventral striatum, an area known to be involved in pleasure.

Functional MRIs have been used to determine high activity in the anterior insula and ventral striatum, both areas that have been associated with feelings of empathy. In one study, when

---

[31] Chow, Denise. (2013). Live Science [blog]. Retrieved from www.livescience.com/37684-narcissistic-personality-disorder-brain-structure.html

physicians felt like they were relieving pain, their brains responded positively. In other words, relieving pain was both positive for the patient and the physician.[32]

Neuroscientists now believe that the information from this research will allow them to design interventions that will change the brain's circuitry. This belief stems from the facts that the brain is malleable, and one's tendency to be empathetic or compassionate is not fixed. Indeed, empathy can be learned.

Active Listening and Empathy

For one to be truly empathetic, one must learn to listen to others. Most of us, including myself, are not good at listening. When we meet someone for the first time, we can't even remember the person's name after the introduction. We are too busy processing the interaction and trying to make a good first impression.

There is a wealth of literature that describes how quickly a physician makes a diagnosis after interviewing a patient for the first time. A recent study[33] revealed that most physicians let patients speak for an average of 22 seconds before they interrupt. The majority of physicians (64% of primary care physicians and 80% of specialists) did not even ask the patient the purpose of his or her visit.

Empathy requires active listening. A physician should orient him- or herself physically to face the patient. Providers should be on the same level, either seated or standing (or kneeling in the instance of a small child). Your body posture

---

[32] (2013). *Molecular Psychiatry*
[33] *Journal of General Internal Medicine* (Jan. 2019, Vol 34, pp. 36-40)

should be open, with shoulders square to the patient, arms at your sides or active, but not folded over your chest. Eye contact should be as close to 100% of the time as possible. It is worth noting that it is difficult to actively listen to someone if you are busy entering data into your computer, walking in and out of the room, concentrating on how *you* look, or what you are going to say next.

When we engage someone in a meaningful way or even in a light conversation, we often concentrate on what our next comment is going to be, not what the speaker is saying. Active listening requires that you acknowledge what the speaker is saying. This would take the form of nodding your head, saying "hmmm," "ah," smiling, and of course, paying attention to the point of what the person is saying and asking questions when you're unclear about what they mean. The visual and audio feedback caregivers provide to patients trying to communicate is critical to the care process. It helps to encourage the speaker by saying "I understand," and "I know how you feel." Paraphrasing what has just been said also opens the conversation and makes it empathetic. Remember, you, as the professional, are responsible for the communication and its meaning. Carol Jones, PhD, noted clinical psychologist and author of *Overcoming Anger,* states that "Empathetic listening can keep you from making erroneous or pejorative judgments. Remember everyone is just trying to survive, doing the best that they can, and you need to recognize their struggle."[34]

---

[34] Jones, Carol. (2004). *Overcoming Anger*. Avon, MA: Adams Media.

Achieving the Correct Balance

An excellent article published in 2014 by Martin Lamothe and others in the *British Medical Journal of Family Practice* entitled "The Combined Role of Empathetic Concern and Perspective Taking in Understanding Burnout in General Practice" discusses the violation of boundaries in practitioners. They write "Good doctor-patient relationships are fundamental for better patient outcomes.[35] It is a meaningful understanding of both the patient's cognitive and affective states; in other words, the patient's knowledge versus feelings."[36] In this context, both empathy and sympathy appear to be crucial components in the doctor-patient relationship. Empathy has been defined as a cognitive (rather than an affective) attribute that involves the practitioner understanding the inner experiences and perspectives of the patient, combined with a capability to communicate this understanding to the patient.'[37] Sympathy has been defined as a predominately emotional state that involves feeling the patient's pain and suffering. The goal of empathy is to know the patient better while the goal of sympathy is to feel the patient's emotions better.[38] It is important to distinguish the two concepts because they may lead to different outcomes.

---

[35] Larson, EB. (2005). Clinical Empathy as Emotional Labor in the Patient-Physician Relationship. *JAMA, 293*, 1100–1106)
[36] Hojat M, et al. (2001). The Jefferson Scale of Physician Empathy. *Educ Psychol Meas, 61,* 349–365
[37] Hojat, M, et al. (2003). Physician Empathy in Medical Education and Practice. *Semin Integr Med, 1*, 25–41
[38] Hojat, M, et al. (2011). Empathetic and Sympathetic Orientations toward Patient Care. *Acad Med, 86*, 989–995.

For example, in a 1991 study, researchers asked physicians to select either the sympathetic response or the empathetic response to a hypothetical patient's misfortune (death of a spouse) and to state their preferences for intubating a hypothetical end-stage lung-disease patient. For each physician, hospital records were retrospectively reviewed to assess the mean number of laboratory tests ordered per clinic patient and the mean duration of cardiopulmonary resuscitations he or she performed before declaring his or her efforts unsuccessful. As hypothesized, physicians who selected the sympathetic option had a greater mean preference for intubation, ordered more laboratory tests per patient in clinic, and performed cardiopulmonary resuscitation for longer periods of time before declaring their efforts unsuccessful than did physicians selecting the empathetic option. It was concluded that a physician's levels of empathy and sympathy have a measurable influence on their practice behavior. Sympathetic physicians used more healthcare resources, and it's worth questioning whether the sympathetic actions actually helped or hurt in the long run.[39]

Some authors believe that empathy leads to personal growth, career satisfaction, and optimal clinical outcomes, while sympathy could be detrimental to objectivity in decision making, and lead to compassion fatigue and burnout.[40] Sympathy can be detrimental if it leads the physician to take his

[39] Nightingale SD, et al. (1991). Sympathy, Empathy and Physician Resource Utilization. *J Ben Intern Med*, 6, 420–423.

emotions home with him or her at the end of the day and, over time, can emotionally wear out the caregiver.

However, being too empathetic toward patients can lead to a myriad of boundary crossings and violations. "Beyond a certain point, empathy could actively hinder a physician's performance and affect medical decision making. Sharing the patient's emotions can lead to empathetic overload and personal distress. Physicians that share patients' emotions may have difficulty maintaining a sense of ownership regarding whose emotions belong to whom. To complement the effect of empathy, professionals need a high level of emotional regulation skills." [41]

Codependency is detrimental to the physician-patient relationship. Codependency is an emotional and behavioral condition that is learned and can be passed down from one generation to another. It is also known as "relationship addiction," because people who are codependent often form or maintain relationships that are one-sided, destructive, and/or abusive. It is usually applied to spouses of alcoholics and substance abusers or those individuals raised in dysfunctional families where codependency was normal. Codependency in a caregiver-patient relationship can be subtle but still have dire consequences for both parties. The physician, nurse, therapist, etc., who has issues of low self-esteem and wants to please all people all the time is in the perfect situation for this problem to evolve. The practitioner who tries to fix problems that the patient is experiencing even though they do not have the

---

[41] Hojat M. (2007). *Empathy in Patient Care*. Berlin, Germany: Springer.

expertise may indicate a tendency toward codependency. The provider who continues to think or obsess about a patient's illness or situation after the provider is removed from the case may also indicate an unhealthy lack of boundaries.

As previously discussed in Chapter 2 on family systems, the child that is reared in an enmeshed family system that is chaotic, closed, and has no boundaries may also produce an adult with poor or absent boundaries. These individuals may have little or no concept of personal space or what is taking place on either side of the equation. The flip side of this is the family that is rigid. These families tend to build walls and barriers instead of healthy boundaries. They isolate themselves physically and emotionally and may show a complete lack of empathy. Codependent families may have a combination of both, which produces adults who have no concept of what healthy empathy or boundaries involve.

Then there are those who swing the opposite way: the narcissists. These individuals routinely violate the boundaries of others due to their almost complete lack of empathy. Individuals who are diagnosed with this disorder meet five of the following criteria:

- Shows a lack of empathy and is unwilling to recognize or identify with the feelings of others
- Has a grandiose sense of self-importance (e.g., exaggerates achievements and talents, expects to be recognized as superior without commensurate achievements)

- Has a sense of entitlement (i.e., unreasonably expects people to show them favorable treatment or automatically comply with his or her expectations)
- Exploits people (i.e., taking advantage of others to achieve his or her own ends).
- Envies others and believes others envy him or her
- Requires excessive admiration
- Demonstrates arrogant or haughty behaviors or attitudes
- Believes that he or she is special and unique and can only be understood by, or should only associate with, other special or high-status people
- Is preoccupied with fantasies of unlimited success, power, brilliance, beauty, or ideal love[42]
- Does not consider the pain they may inflict on others; simply put, they do not care about thoughts, emotions, or feelings of others. Their world revolves around them.

The Endgame of Empathy

Empathy should benefit the patient and the provider. Empathy can be exhibited in many ways, but the key is that the patient, client, staff, or family member recognizes that you are "on their side." This could be simply listening a little longer, saying you understand, or maintaining eye contact instead of looking down at your computer. It could be answering the same

---

[42] (2014). BPD Central [blog]. Retrieved from
https:/bpdecentral.com/narcissistic-disorder/hallmarks-of-npd

question twice without an exasperated look on your face. It might be patting someone on the shoulder or holding the hand of an elderly patient who has just lost her husband. It could be accepting a hug from a grateful parent. All of these encounters require knowledge of boundaries. Some are crossings, but remember that boundaries are contextual, and our humanity is critical to empathetic and effective care.

In his study cited above, Bergland postulates that there are ways an individual can start to alter his or her neural pathways to increase empathy. He suggests "mindfulness meditation" in which a person takes a few moments every day to have good thoughts about the self and others. Oxytocin, which is called the feel-good neurochemical, is released when you pet a dog, give a gift, or meditate while focusing on others. It is produced in the hypothalamus and secreted by the posterior lobe of the pituitary gland. He also suggests physical exercise to release epinephrine. Seeking or studying disagreeable situations may help you avoid overreacting or feeling overly empathetic to the point that it is unhealthy. Lastly, he recommends volunteering to help others in order to help cultivate feelings of empathy.

As in most things, moderation is a worthwhile target for empathy. An overabundance or lack of empathy may cause patients to accuse a practitioner of boundary violations. Understanding empathy and its ramifications is an absolute must for maintaining proper boundaries.

Take Aways
- Empathy increases patient satisfaction and clinical outcomes.

- Empathy improves the physician's and provider's wellbeing.
- Empathy is a learned skill.
- Be aware of co-dependency in your professional relationships.
- Ask unscripted questions of your patients.
- Practice "active listening."

Chapter 5:
The Ethics of it All

Ethical behavior refers to the choices you make when no one else is looking, whether at home, in public, or in the practice setting. Unfortunately, there is no black-and-white way to define what behavior is considered ethical or unethical. Ethical behavior hinges on multiple factors, including context, culture, professional standards, moral guidelines, family backgrounds and values, and religious beliefs. By nature, ethics are subjective: what may appear ethical to you may or may not be considered ethical to someone else. Therefore, your internal compass is what really counts.

As practitioners, we don't always have the privilege to determine what is ethical or not. That is why most fiduciary bodies of medicine, law, clergy and many others have ethical standards for their membership. In fact, most of these organizations have the power to remove members if they fail to meet certain criteria.

Given the nebulous nature of ethics, all of us could benefit from what Peggy Noonan writing in the *Wall Street Journal* calls an "Ethical Fitbit that could report at the end of each day that you have taken 12,304 constructive steps, some uphill, or 3,297 destructive ones and appropriate action is warranted." Many times, it is just not obvious that we have strayed from an ethical path. Rather, an ethical violation doesn't become a problem until it is a problem (and in the case of medical practitioners, it's often a big problem).

The goal of this chapter is to help define ethical standards as they pertain to physician-patient boundaries and help you realize how ethical violations may affect your professional relationships and your professional standing.

Don Berwick, MD, writes for *JAMA* that moral (ethical) choices sometimes arrive with drama, but most do not. Most come unannounced, silent on arrival, as Carl Sandburg's poem *Fog* describes a fog rolling in on "little cat feet."

The foundation of ethical boundaries in healthcare was established almost three thousand years ago. The Hippocratic Oath, written in the fourth century BC by Hippocrates and possibly other contributors, remains the foundation for medical ethics. It may be even more relevant today than it was when it was written. The classic version has the physician swearing an oath to the Greek gods Asclepius, Hygieia, and Panaceia. It starts with promising to share their knowledge and experience with others as they have benefited from others' instruction. They swear to help the sick according to their ability and judgment and will keep the patient from harm and injustice (First: Do no harm). Furthermore "whatever houses I may visit, I will come for the benefit of the sick, remaining free of all intentional injustice, of all mischief and in particular of sexual relations with both female and male persons, be they free or slaves. What I may see or hear in the course of their treatment or even outside of the treatment in regard to the life of men, which on no account one must spread abroad, I will keep to myself holding such things shameful to be spoken about." The oath finishes with a recommendation or resolution if you do not abide by it. "If I fulfill this oath and do not violate it, may it be granted to me to enjoy life and art, being honored with fame among all men for all time to come; if I transgress it and swear falsely, may the opposite of all this be my lot."

Biomedical ethics encompass every tricky aspect of healthcare, including abortion, euthanasia, human research, use of technology, capital punishment, and use of genetic engineering. For the purposes of this chapter, however, we will concentrate on boundaries pertaining to the physician-patient relationship.

Five moral theories have been developed over the centuries for determining ethical behavior. Most likely, none of us will mentally review these before making a decision or action involving ethics, but a general background knowledge will be beneficial. An understanding will not only help us with our internal ethical compass but will help explain how others view our behavior. The five moral theories are:

- Deontology
- Consequentialism
- Justice theory
- Virtue ethics
- Care ethics

Deontology views moral life in the context of duties, obligations, and what is right. Basically, a deontologist believes that an action that has an honorable intention and is done for the sake of duty is correct regardless of the consequences of that action. It commands that we act in ways consistent with reason and logic, regardless of our own wishes, desires, emotions, or circumstances. Respect for your fellow human beings is the central value.

Consequentialism essentially states that an action or rule is right if it is likely to produce more good consequences than bad. Consequentialism is based on utilitarianism, which theorizes that what is important is happiness and pleasure along with the avoidance of pain. The utilitarian is directed to consider all the options, consider all those whose happiness will be affected, assign a value to each person's happiness in the equation, add up the total happiness and subtract the unhappiness, and ultimately choose the option with the most happiness.

Justice theory supposes that each of us gets what we deserve or are owed. Justice theory should not be confused with equality. Equality means that everyone gets the same thing. Fairness, the basis for justice theory, means that everyone's needs are met individually. Aristotle, in the 4th Century BC, was the architect behind justice theory. He sought to provide a framework for judging right and wrong in a way that treats everyone fairly and respects individuals' rights. In providing someone their rights, others may need to act positively or negatively toward that person. For example, if you have an inherent right to privacy, then others have a moral duty not to spy on you, read your mail, or reveal your health records. Rights and duties are linked.

Virtue ethics assumes that an individual can become a good person. It is not based on actions, but on the person. Aristotle defined virtue as the excellence of the human soul. Today, we consider courage, honesty, generosity, and friendliness to be virtues. Virtue ethics do not provide a path to follow but assumes that if we are virtuous, we will do the right thing for the right reason. In other words, the virtuous person will behave in a thoughtful, compassionate, and sensitive manner.

Care ethics postulates that women have a unique ability to provide care. It assumes most nurses are female and physicians are male, which we know today is incorrect and not relevant. It is a feminist approach that argues that we are not independent or objective, but rather born into a web of relationships of family, friends, and colleagues that explain or determine the context of our lives. Some nursing theorists posit that nurses have a unique trait of caring for others and advocating for patients.

How Ethics Applies to Medicine

Tim Beauchamp, PhD, and James Childress, PhD, presented their four principles for biomedical ethics in their 1977 book *Principles of Biomedical Ethics,* which has since become a foundational text in the medical field. Their position was that most ethical decisions in medicine are urgent and require a rapid response. The four principles are autonomy, beneficence, nonmaleficence, and justice.

The principle of **autonomy** basically states that each competent person has the right to make medical decisions that affect his or her life. Because each person has different values, beliefs, and preferences, each person should get to decide for him- or herself. This is contradictory to the age-old history of paternalism, or the "rule of the father," which essentially allowed physicians to make decisions without input from the patient. Informed consent and advance directives are now the rule and not the exception.

The second principle is that of **beneficence** or "doing good" for our patients. This is a given in the practice of medicine and other healing professions. In healthcare, we are all charged with the duty to make lives better, improve patients' situations, and make people well again when it is possible.

The third principle, **nonmaleficence,** is the corollary to beneficence. In other words, if we are not able to "do good," then we at least should do no harm. Harm is a subjective term and is dependent again on individual values, beliefs, and wishes. What is harmful to some would not be considered harmful to others.

The fourth principle is **justice** and simply means that all patients should be treated justly, fairly, and equally in similar circumstances.

All of these theories and principles are worthy of reflection, but as David Chambers, PhD, writes, "Our temptations are educable: we respond instantly and naturally to common occurring circumstances. The time to get good at ethics is not when confronted with temptation, but by systematically reviewing policies to identify structural ethical traps."[43]

Healthcare providers and other professionals, regardless of their degree or license, are held to a high ethical standard. The power differential demands it. The American Medical Association addresses it in its *Principles of Medical Ethics*:

---

[43] Journal of the American College of Dentists, 78:3, 2011.

"The practice of medicine, and its embodiment in the clinical encounter between a patient and a physician, is fundamentally a moral activity that arises from the imperative to care for patients and to alleviate suffering. The relationship between a patient and a physician is based on trust, which gives rise to physicians' ethical responsibility to place patients' welfare above the physician's own self-interest or obligations to others, to use sound medical judgment on patients' behalf, and to advocate for their patients' welfare."

Article 1.2.1 states "Treating oneself or a member on one's own family poses several challenges to physicians, including concerns about professional objectivity, patient autonomy and informed consent...In general, physicians should not treat themselves or members of their own families."

There are exceptions in emergency situations or possibly for short-term problems. It is a slippery slope. Treating your own child's sinus infection with appropriate antibiotics becomes troublesome, if not illegal, when you also prescribe a controlled substance for pain management. A dentist who removes a family member's abscessed tooth seems innocuous, but if the practitioner prescribes narcotics during the course of treatment, then several boundaries have been crossed and/or violated. Treating outside of your specialty is also an ethical no-no. A pathologist should not routinely prescribe anti-hypertensives or contraceptives for her friends and neighbors. A plastic and reconstructive surgeon should probably leave the practice of managing acute ketoacidosis to others.

Establishing and maintaining professional boundaries and professional ethics are two sides of the same coin. They cannot be separated. If you have a license, then you automatically possess the power in the professional relationship. The power is derived from real and perceived factors. The medical legacy, the title of doctor, the attainment of an elite education coupled with your ego and abilities firmly establishes the power differential. You are likewise bound by your oath to practice your art and science as well as your employer's or medical staff's code of conduct. The approach you take when interacting with your patients, their families, your staff, other staff members, students, trainees, and colleagues all determine how you exercise this power. Curbside consults, bartering for professional services, granting discounts or free care to some but not all, making special arrangements for staff or influential patients are all examples of misusing your power.

Using your white coat and stethoscope to attract romantic attention in the workplace is another example that violates ethical standards. Patients, clients, nurses, students, staff, sales representatives, and anyone else you have a professional relationship with should all be in your "no-fly" zone. It is impractical to think that professionals will not be attracted to any of the people they work with, but as stated previously, it is not a problem until it is a problem. Again, the AMA *Principles of Medical Ethics* is very clear: "Sexual relationships between a medical trainee or supervisee, even if consensual, is not acceptable, regardless of the degree of separation in any situation."

Ethics and Romance

We can't talk about ethical behavior without touching on the possibility that practitioners may be accused of sexual misconduct at some point in their careers. There are two sides, sometimes three, to every story of sexual misconduct. The AMA *Code of Medical Ethics* is clear and murky at the same time regarding this issue. Opinion 9.1.1 states:

"Romantic or sexual interactions between physicians and patients that occur concurrently with the patient-physician relationship are unethical. Such interactions detract from the goals of the patient-physician relationship and may exploit the vulnerability of the patient, compromise the physician's ability to make objective judgments about the patient's healthcare, and ultimately may be detrimental to the patient's wellbeing. A physician must terminate the patient-physician relationship before initiating a dating, romantic, or sexual relationship with a patient. Likewise, sexual or romantic relationships between a physician and a former patient maybe unduly influenced by the previous physician-patient relationship. Sexual or romantic relationships with former patients are unethical if the physician uses or exploits trust, knowledge, emotions, or influence derived for the previous professional relationship, or if a romantic relationship would otherwise foreseeably harm the individual. In keeping with a physician's ethical obligations to avoid inappropriate behavior, a physician who has reason to believe that nonsexual, nonclinical contact with a patient may be perceived as or may lead to romantic or sexual contact should be avoided."

A consensual relationship simply cannot exist when the power differential and the vulnerability of the patient or client is considered. Context is critical here, but of all the boundary crossings or violations, this one carries the greatest risk for both the physician and the patient. Licensing boards take a guilty-until-proven-innocent stance with regard to allegations of sexual misconduct, and if the charges are substantiated or proven, then it is viewed as a complete failure of medical ethics. In that case, the practitioner's license to practice is in jeopardy. Board actions are based on frequency and severity. Sexual misconduct allegations tend to place individuals at the top of the list very quickly.

Practicing physicians may view a sexual misconduct allegation somewhat differently. A Medscape survey published in December 2014 written by Leslie Kane, MA, illustrates that a growing number of physicians are ok with what others consider inappropriate relationships. The survey asked practitioners "Is it acceptable to be involved in a romantic or sexual relationship with a patient?" In 2010 and again in 2014, 1% answered that it is acceptable. However, in 2010, 12% stated yes, but not until at least six months have passed since the patient stopped being a patient. In 2014, 22% of respondents gave that same response. Similarly, in 2010, 83% answered the question with a flat no, but by 2014, only 68% did. Some of the added comments were instructive as well, such as "Love should not be denied, but you should immediately and formally sever the patient-physician relationship." One physician went so far as to say, "You should give time for feelings to cool off and see if the attraction was simply a result of the power imbalance inherent in most patient relationships."

In a 2002 article on Managedcare.com, Michael Victoroff, MD, wrote, "A physician-patient romance deserves a sophisticated and courageous ethical analysis. We need to rise above the cynical view that love cannot exist, and sex must be abusive and transient between people with power disparities. Our professional standards are perfectly rational and make fine common sense. But love obeys different rules."

These findings and comments are all well and good and are definitely worthy of consideration, but many factors are at play. For example, one must consider the intentions and motives on both sides of the power differential and the risks versus benefits in any romantic workplace relationship. If a relationship ends well, no harm no foul, but if it goes south, then allegations, lawsuits, loss of employment, and board actions may follow. There is some logic, of course, in the two parties discussing the relationship once the professional relationship has ceased. But it must be noted that severing the physician-patient relationship is harder in some disciplines than others. For example, internal medicine, family practice, mental health, and obstetrics and gynecology practitioners see certain patients often and get to know them intimately, providing fertile soil for romantic relationships to bloom. The close connection also makes ending the professional relationship more difficult than, say, a urologist who sees a patient twice a year. The majority of participants in our boundaries classes are from these specialties.

Boundary violations and ethics are welded together. Everyone has to determine and develop their own ethical guidelines for their own boundaries. Something as simple as a hug can be misconstrued. The goal for this entire book is for the reader to have a full understanding of how maintaining boundaries can affect your entire practice and career going forward.

Take-Aways
- We all could use an "ethical Fit-bit."
- Ethics are always situational.
- The professional is always responsible for the ethical decision-making and behavior.
- Ethics are both objective and subjective.
- Ethical distinctions are usually blurry and not well defined.
- Many times, the recipient of the ethical encounter determines the outcome.

Chapter 6:
Healthy Sexual Boundaries

As in the previous chapters discussing ethics and empathy, any discussion of sexual boundaries must touch on a series of complex social and emotional human responses. In this chapter, we will cover the intimacy inherent in providing healthcare and a practitioner's possible misuse of power; the many definitions of masculine and feminine roles and the vulnerabilities created therein; as well as the sensual perception of touch, regardless of whether it is intended to be sexual in nature. Finally, we will discuss nonverbal cues and messages about sensuality and sexuality in the clinical setting that can lead to boundary violations.

The Sexual Journey

The sexual journey begins at birth when a baby is deemed a boy or a girl based on anatomy. Consciously and unconsciously, this gender assignment determines how the toddler and child dresses, society's expectations of how he or she chooses toys and games, and the development of his or her gender identity. Being a boy or a girl relies far less on physical anatomy, but rather on the child's perception of the self as male or female. This gender identity eventually develops into a gender role, the composite of all the thoughts, actions, and feelings that make up the child's portrayal of a man or a woman. A wide variety of thoughts, emotions, and actions make up a gender role, and it is a major factor in determining how the child will act in relationships.

With the help of cultural, familial, social, and other influences, children begin to divide themselves into the two major gender roles: boys and girls. With the onset of puberty, the expression of gender roles becomes complex, and children start constructing their own ideas about boundaries.

Initially, the development of gender identity and gender roles are internalizations of what a child observes in the environment. However, some aspects of this development are innate, nature rather than nurture. For example, even if a child's parents avoid violence in the media and discourage combative play, the child, male or female, may still feel the strong urge to pick up a stick and turn it into a sword. Little objective clarity exists to help us understand how and where children develop these assumed modes of play.

The boundaries between boys and girls that develop in early childhood may become somewhat rigid (think of the outdated term "cooties") but then, possibly through peer pressure, begin to dissolve. Adolescents are typically cumbersome and even shy when learning how to approach the opposite sex. As the social boundaries begin to dissolve, the physical boundaries are initially intimidating, but eventually become enticing. At first, figuring out how to hold hands appears monumental, but yields to an arm around each other or dancing, or, eventually, the magic of a first kiss. Movies and literature would tell us that something magical happens with each of these events, and it is supposed to draw us into relationships. The reality is that the process of negotiating more and more intimate boundaries is often fraught with fear, pain, disappointment and, hopefully, laughable moments.

In the background of the adolescent's struggle to create adult-like relationships exists conflicting messages. Hormones are driving the car quickly toward sexuality, yet teens are often encouraged to put on the brakes. Often, our somewhat puritanical culture sends the message that sexual urges should be ignored because sex itself is dirty. A fortunate child is one who is taught early on that sex is one part of healthy relationships and intimacy.

If coming into one's own sexuality wasn't complicated enough, society sends young adults confusing and exaggerated messages. For example, losing one's virginity is often considered a goal (or even a right) for males, while teen girls are either considered someone else's prize or marked with shame. For a male, losing his virginity is a badge of honor when, in reality, nothing changes physically for a male when he has sex. Historically speaking, however, virginity is the ancient mark of ownership for females. A girl's father owns her until she is "taken in marriage." Provided she is a virgin, then her husband receives an "intact" prize to marry. Sexual boundary violations echo this notion that purity is a virtue. Thus, for the recipient of a boundary violation, particularly a female, the violation becomes a negative mark on her conscience and the feeling that the offender has taken something from her.

Is Sex the End of The Sexual Journey?

The fundamental components of sexuality are intimacy, sensuality, and sexual behavior. Much of the focus on boundaries has traditionally been on the last component. However, as we grow our awareness of the issue, we can take a broader view. To fully examine boundaries, let's start with a look at intimacy and sensuality.

Intimacy

We are constantly in relationships with people on some level. Driving on the freeway, our relationships with the other drivers are distant and disconnected. When we enter a parking lot, we have constraints and must interact more directly by, for example, stopping to let someone cross the street. As we move toward the entrance of the office, store, or apartment building, we enter into relationships with passersby that are more related and interactive but do not require communication or even eye contact. When we walk into a meeting or other gathering of peers or community members, we are met with more interactive relationships that require moving into various levels of intimacy. Our sense of personal space is affected by the number of people in the room. Rarely do we have much verbal discussion of how to negotiate claiming our own space and establishing our position; rather this is often done with body language and a strong sense of needing to maintain an appropriate distance. As conversation develops, we carefully start to navigate the intellectual and emotional space of the other people in the room. If this is a social setting and not business, we may pick one or a few people to spend most of our time interacting with. Once we begin to work within a four-foot radius, we have invited people into our personal space and, whether conscious or not, our relationship becomes more intimate. Other than shaking hands, physical contact during a conversation represents moving into the closest interpersonal space. Many people are uncomfortable with others moving into that space.

In contrast, many of the essential functions of healthcare interactions require invading the personal space of a patient through physical contact. On one level, the patient agreeing to step into that interaction, to some degree, defines his or her willingness to allow this transgression of boundaries. However, a wise and caring practitioner can only help the interaction proceed comfortably by reassuring the patient, asking permission to touch a certain area, and demonstrating an understanding of the process.

Using the terms "intimate" or "intimacy" in a professional relationship is complicated. The term is not inherently linked with sex or sexuality; rather, it may just mean "close," "vulnerable," or "revealing." For example, one can dine with a friend in an intimate venue or have an intimate conversation with a sibling. A patient showing her physician a part of her body she doesn't show anyone else can feel intimate but not be related at all to sex or sexual feelings. When sex is equated with intimacy, the concept of boundaries is omitted. In other words, when one person in a relationship equates intimacy with sex and the other doesn't, boundaries are bound to be violated.

Part of the art and power of providing all levels of healthcare is the fact that it is a very intimate interaction. When a human being allows another human being to touch them, whether this is implied or under formal consent, it is a level of trust to which other people in that patient's life may not have access.

For instance, a pregnant woman from another culture may present to an emergency room with an issue that requires a pelvic exam to determine whether she needs to be transferred to hospital that provides obstetrics. The only physician available is male, but in that woman's culture, allowing a man besides her husband to examine, touch, or view her genitalia may have dire consequences. However, that culture also forbids her to contradict a man. If we add to this the complication of a language barrier, she may not be able to communicate this to the physician and may experience the exam with much anxiety. Furthermore, the urgency of the situation and the climate in the emergency room may not allow the physician to even consider asking the patient culturally sensitive questions. The job just has to get done. This example serves as a reminder for healthcare providers at all levels to honor the sheer intimacy of what we do and the impact that can have on the individual.

Masculinity, Femininity, and Vulnerability

The norms of gender, sex, and power are, in great part, developed and controlled on a cultural level. Terrence Real, in his book *How Can I Get Through to You*, describes American culture as a psychological patriarchy which has three basic rules. Roughly paraphrased, they are:
1. Masculine is more valuable than feminine.
2. Feminine must be treated with scorn and contempt.
3. The dynamic of the scorn and contempt must be kept secret [and denied].

We see these rules at play in our society every day: males are often paid more to do the same job as females. Many insults are related to feminine qualities, female body parts, female roles, and derogatory terms. Boys who are not athletic or strong are often criticized for being "girlish." Likewise, girls who are more athletic, stronger, and more competitive are often criticized as lacking feminine qualities.

In reading this, your first reflex may be to claim that our society has moved forward and these things are not as true as they used to be. Unfortunately, this denial is rule number three in Real's psychological patriarchy. In the example previously of the male physician in the emergency room, one might theorize that the male physician has the right to initiate the examination without asking for the patient's permission. Similarly, in keeping with the second rule, the nurse or assistant who asks the woman if she is uncomfortable being examined by a male may be chastised for overstepping her role or is silenced. The reader is invited at this point to re-read the above example, envisioning the physician, nurse or assistant, and patient as the opposite gender. Any differences that arise may well be evidence of this hidden set of rules.

The concept of the psychological patriarchy adds a new layer of complexity to the patient-provider relationship that providers need to be sensitive to. For example, the "#MeToo" movement has highlighted the impact of Real's psychological patriarchy. Victims (mainly women) of crimes, assaults, and harassment are speaking out after decades of being silenced by the patriarchy. As a result of this movement and society's growing dissatisfaction with the status quo, what a practitioner might have seen as routine years ago might be considered a violation today.

Nonverbal Parts of Sexuality

We often think that sexuality is overt and aggressive and that the power differential between patient and provider is abundantly clear. But even if a provider does not send any direct sexual messages or does not flaunt his or her power, he or she can still violate boundaries through non-verbal cues.

Silence can be a powerful non-verbal assertion of power. Whether the silence is the pause to reflect, the quiet of not knowing the answer, or the plain refusal to speak, the power is present. If we don't take the time to reflect how our silence affects the patient, we can harm the relationship. Beyond the silence, every patient hears the sigh, the chuckle or smirk we think is silent, or the quiet "harrumph" of frustration. Feeling like the powerless person in the relationship, the patient may not be able to challenge or counter the physician's silence. The responsibility for paying attention to these subtle gestures lies with those of us to whom the patients have entrusted their well-being. Patients watch each gesture, movement, and facial expression in an effort to guess what is happening. They are reading you.

The most impactful nonverbal component of sexuality is body language. Body position, touch, and proximity are all tools that can be used to connect with the patient or maintain a boundary. However, the wild card is the patient's interpretation. He or she may feel intimidated by a practitioner's actions or may see them as welcomed gestures. The remedy is to be aware of not only your own non-verbal gestures, but also the patient's. If moving closer leads the patient to pull away or shrink, then back off. If a provider notices her arms are folded across her chest, simply relaxing the arms to the sides may bring about a notable shift in the patient's demeanor. Another good rule is to ask simple permission before touching the patient. "May I hold your hand?" A simple question and a pause may change the whole dynamic of the encounter. Always keep in mind that the patient's language may say "yes" but the body may clearly say "no."

No matter what you, as the provider, intend, you always run the risk of a patient misinterpreting a gesture. In the fear, pain, and vulnerability of being in need, a patient may misconstrue your gentle hand laid on his or her shaking hand as a seductive invitation. Even though that is not the intention, the patient may be enamored with the provider's power and experience a vastly different meaning. A friendly conversation that has nothing to do with the visit may be perceived as a budding relationship. The fast track to a boundary violation ends in a complaint to the employer or licensing agent.

Sexuality is in our DNA and affects every interaction we have with other humans. Becoming aware of the power differential, the gender divide, and our own body language is the key to maintaining healthy boundaries and providing safe and effective care to both men and women.

Take Aways
- When sex is equated with intimacy, the concept of boundaries is omitted.

- The male/female roles may well be a hidden set or rules.
- Pay attention to body language. It speaks louder than words.
- Always be aware of the power differential.

Chapter 7:
Separating the Problems from the Issues with Sexual Boundary Violations

In the previous chapter, we discussed healthy sexual boundaries and sexuality. Understanding your own sexuality and what healthy sexual boundaries should look like is vital to identifying sexual boundary violations. Sexual harassment, abuse, and inappropriate relationships always leave a trail of disappointment, anger, and shame. The patient, nurse, trainee, or coworker who has been abused nearly always feels overwhelmed with shame and fears that he or she will be blamed for the behavior or incident. Many healthcare organizations, hospitals, clinics, and regulatory boards have an inadequate or broken reporting mechanism that tends to favor the physician. An 2016 investigation by the *Atlanta Journal-Constitution* identified more than 2,400 cases of physicians around the country who had "sexually assaulted" patients[44]. The investigation revealed that half of these physicians were still licensed to practice medicine.

Sexual misconduct is concentrated in (but not limited to) the specialties of family medicine, psychiatry, internal medicine, and obstetrics and gynecology.[45][46] An analysis of 101 cases of

---

[44] Teegardin, C, Robbin, D, et al , License to Betray, 2016
[45] Enbom JA, Parshley P, et al, A Follow up evaluation of sexual misconduct complaints: the Oregon Board of Medical Examiners, 1998 through 2002. Am J Obstet Gynecol, 2004, 1642-50.
[46] Kohatsu ND, Gould D, et al, Characteristics associated with physician discipline: a case-control study, Arch Intern Med 2004, 653-8

sexual abuse of patients by physicians revealed that all of the abusers were male, most (92%) were 39 years old or older, and that 72% of the cases involved a non-consensual sexual relationship. Patients were consistently examined without a chaperone present (85%), and in non-academic settings (94%).[47]

When Does Behavior Become Problematic?

Given the frightening statistics and the dire consequences to both parties (potential loss of license for the physician and a lifetime of shame and the emotional and sometimes legal aftermath of trauma for the abused), we must ask why practitioners engage in this behavior at all? For some practitioners with a poor understanding of healthy boundaries, crossing sexual boundaries becomes a slippery slope. If the gentle hand on the shoulder was okay, then the hand on the knee must be ok, and if the hand on the knee is okay, the hug must be okay, and on and on, creating a snowball effect. The practitioner continues to stretch the boundaries until one day, he or she is faced with a very big problem.

When it comes human behavior, there is a saying, "The problem is rarely the issue," which means that we sometimes focus so much on the problem, such as sexual boundary violations, that we miss the importance of identifying the behaviors that created the issue, namely poor boundaries that invite harmful behaviors. In this section we will discuss two

---

[47] Dubois JM, Walsh HA, et al, Sexual violation of patients by physicians: a mixed-methods, exploratory analysis of 101 cases, Sex Abuse, 2019, 503-23.

problems that are often the result of much deeper issues: problematic sexual behavior on the part of the practitioner and patients with extremely poor boundaries and destructive motivation, sometimes negatively labeled "seductive patients."

In the *Journal of Sexual Addiction and Compulsion*, Bill Herring, LSCW and certified sex addition therapist, presents a neutral framework for identifying when behavior is problematic. This framework describes sexual behavior as problematic if it consistently:

- Conflicts with a person's commitments and/or
- Conflicts with a person's values and/or
- Conflicts with a person's self-control and/or
- Results in negative consequences and/or
- Lacks fundamental sexual responsibility

These five categories each yield a question to consider when addressing any problematic components of a person's ongoing destructive sexual behavior:

- Commitments: Are you keeping your promises? What did you agree to with your license or certification (think of the Hippocratic Oath)?
- Values: Are you OK with what you are doing based on your internal values?
- Control: Are you in control of yourself and acting by choice?
- Consequences: Would you be worried if you had been under video observation?
- Responsibility: Are you protecting others, adhering to the adage to "First, do no harm?"

What Happens When Boundaries are Broken by Problematic Behavior?

From a regulatory and institutional perspective, the usual first response is to remove the person engaging in problematic behavior. However, this book is about both prevention and intervention. Behind the broken boundaries lies a human who can learn, grow, and be productive. There are those who are truly harmful and should be removed from a position of power. It is up to the professional assessment team within each institution to identify the individuals who are truly unable to change their behavior and return to work. The recommendations for those few individuals are clear and career-ending.

As with any situation that seems problematic, whether regarding sexual boundaries or other violations, the first task is to identify the problem. This involves looking in detail at the event that led to a complaint or a concern on the part of an employer. This type of assessment is typically done by a professional assessment team, which includes psychiatrists, psychologists, nurses, substance abuse treatment providers, and specially trained peers in the professional group. It typically occurs over three to five days and involves psychological testing; drug testing by both body fluids and, if indicated, hair follicle testing; forensic interviews; and, in some cases, polygraph. The team discusses their findings and makes a series of recommendations, which are usually binding and are aimed at returning the person to functional status through education, monitoring, supervisory and peer support, and many other facets of rehabilitation. This chapter does not define any single process of assessment nor delves into the details of treatment—those specifics are determined by the institution and the scenario.

For a significant majority, the goal of the assessment and subsequent treatment is to return the practitioner to work without fear on the part of the caregiver, the institution for whom they work, or the patient. While the strict standards of Physician Health Programs are good ones to apply to sexuality in general, they are valid references for general professional behavior. Looking at all the elements that led up to and were involved in this specific boundary-breaking event is essential to separating out truly *dangerous* behavior from the many categories of *problematic* behavior.

The professional assessment team looks for answers to the following types of questions:

- Is this a singular occurrence, or is it part of a pattern of behavior both on the job and in the practitioner's personal life?
- To what extent did the occurrence require planning and preparation?
- What is the individual's willingness and ability to tell different interviewers a relatively consistent story that not only makes sense, but also matches the victim's report?
- To what degree is the individual willing to allow the evaluation team to obtain information from peers, family members, and other corroborative sources?

- Are there issues such as substance use, legal history, or undisclosed information about past behaviors that raise concern?

The goal of this line of questioning is to separate people with patterns of disruptive, illegal, and other predatory behaviors from those who are assessed for problematic sexual behavior and boundary violations. The assessment and treatment of individuals with predatory patterns of behavior is much more complex than will be addressed in this book. Suffice it to say that these persons are highly unlikely to ever return to the profession in which the typically egregious boundary violation occurred.

Instead, this book focuses on patterns of behavior that, while they do cross and violate boundaries, do not indicate progressive behavior. We will focus on people who have patterns of behavior that are impulsive, minimally complex in their planning and, frequently, incidental or accidental in their process. These individuals are often amenable to education and rehabilitation.

Boundary Crossings and Boundary Transgressions

Early boundary crossings are crossings of traditional boundaries that are intended to be helpful and are welcomed by the patient. In the field of mental health, a typical guideline is that physical contact with patients, particularly hugs and extended hand-to-hand or hand-to-arm contact, are not a part of usual treatment. However, there are many times where these types of gestures can be grounding and helpful to a patient. Likewise, a disorientated patient in a nursing home may respond better to a gentle hand on the arm, or even an arm around the shoulders, to help guide them back to their room than to forceful verbal redirection. These types of interactions are just as likely to raise the eyebrows of employers as they are to receive commendation from family members and other support staff. So, where is the line when it comes to touching? Healthcare institutions need to establish expectations clearly and specifically. Any boundary crossing needs to be carefully thought out in terms of what it means to the provider and what it may mean to the patient, and one is wise to always err on the side of caution.

Boundary crossings are any kind of contact or statement that causes the patient discomfort. These may not be overt insults or direct physical contact, and the practitioner may have had the best of intentions; however the discomfort is in the eyes of the patient or recipient. While terms of endearment such as "Honey" or "Dear" are often intended to be affectionate, engaging, and welcoming, there are people for whom these words are offensive and patronizing. Consider a hand placed on the shoulder. To one person, it may feel like a gesture of comfort or assurance, whereas to another person with a history of physical trauma or abuse, it may be uncomfortable or even a trigger. The provider has no way of knowing a lot of these details and may only find out that they have crossed a line when a complaint is filed and the supervisor or employer is involved.

When boundary violations are random and unintentional and the provider's intent to do no harm is verified by peers, family, and supervisors, the practitioner may simply need additional education (online or in person) and supervisory monitoring. If substance abuse is a potential issue, random drug screens may be recommended for a period of time. In addition, restricted or supervised patient contact may also be a part of the rehabilitation process, not as a punishment but as an opportunity to observe and reinforce positive behaviors and highlight behaviors that may be of concern while not yet problematic. Practitioners with mental health issues, such as depression, anxiety disorders, and post-traumatic stress disorder will need more intense rehabilitation, including psychiatric assessment and a recommendation to start therapy. Rarely does an assessment team actually provide that level of treatment; rather, to maintain its unbiased position, the team would refer the practitioner to an outside therapist or counselor.

Assessment and treatment

Once a boundary violation has occurred in which there is harm or potential harm to a patient, we must assume that the practitioner's clinical judgement is impaired to some degree. Whether this is a single incident or a subtle pattern, something has led that practitioner to willingly violate boundaries and risk harm to the patient. These types of assessments are more difficult and more detailed and usually involve more extensive treatment. The treatment for compulsive sexual violations requires a clear understanding of all of the factors that lead the practitioner to ignore his or her own core values and the potential consequences of his or her actions. In the vast majority of these cases, by the time the assessment is done, the practitioner's license has been placed on hold or suspended, depending on the guidelines of the licensing agency. The practitioner is unable to work until the institution and the licensing body have some level of assurance that the practitioner can safely return to practice. Naturally, the treatment process takes time. Not only does the treatment team want to understand the underlying issues that led the practitioner to violate sexual boundaries in the first place, but also the potential for it happening again and whether the practitioner is truly dedicated to changing his or her behavior.

Once the practitioner has started treatment and identified the underlying issues that led to the violation (past trauma, family history, mental illness, etc.), he or she must develop a plan for self-care before considering returning to work. A self-care plan may involve group and individual therapy, as well as professional support groups, which many hospitals are adopting as a way to prevent burnout. Assessment teams frequently suggest that a practitioner stay in multiple modes of therapy for as little as six weeks to as long as six months or more. Assessment teams will also recommend that a practitioner set and reach specific measurable goals before ending therapeutic treatment. The practitioner is encouraged to set these goals, rather than the assessment team.

At the end of treatment, the licensing board will review the practitioners progress toward his or her treatment goals and make a decision about whether the practitioner can safely return to work. Occasionally, the licensing board will request a second independent evaluation to review the initial evaluation, the course of treatment, and the practitioner's progress before allowing the individual to return to work. Once the practitioner returns to work, the licensing agency will usually require several types of monitoring. Colleagues may be asked to monitor the practitioner's performance, and the practitioner may be subject to drug screenings and mental-health check-ins. This kind of monitoring has been successful in physician health programs which, as noted previously, have an 86% to 93% success rate at five years. We do remind readers that these are very broad scenarios and do not address all of the assessment and treatment options available.

Healthy Boundaries Help Define Healthy Sexuality and Behavior

When sexual boundaries have been violated and problematic sexual behaviors have been identified, the goal of assessment, treatment, and recovery is to develop a personal definition of healthy sexual behavior.

One of the best measures of appropriate behavior is **consistency**. Asking "Would I do this for every patient I encounter today?" is a very good start. If the answer is "No," then asking for guidance or supervision would be an essential action. Even in special cases, asking "Would I do this for every case like this?" can provide valuable insight into your motivation and potential secondary gain. Consistency provides reproducible behavior across multiple situations that may vary in detail but demand the same level of professional response.

For instance, it is very rare for a psychiatrist to make a house call. However, I can think of a 90+ year old patient who was placed on home hospice care. He asked if I would come to visit. Having seen him for several years, mainly for medication, but always for supportive therapy in the aging and dying process, I sensed that he had a specific issue to process. I asked his family to discuss a home visit with the patient and amongst themselves and make sure they were all comfortable. They were aware that I would maintain the level of confidentiality with which they were familiar. I came to the conclusion that I would make this accommodation for any patient in that age group with a terminal condition and a supportive family. It was a very rewarding and valuable experience for me, for the patient, and for the family.

Boundaries must not only be consistent, but must maintain congruence, defined as agreement, harmony, or compatibility. Congruence must begin with our professional performance being in harmony with our core values, moral senses, and life goals. While relying on consistency for measure, being internally congruent allows us to also be in harmony with the institutional boundaries and regulatory guidelines of the organization.

Remaining congruent internally and institutionally allows us to face challenges, such as difficult patients, complaints (especially those we feel are not valid), and other confrontations with peace of mind. When I can honestly say that I am consistent in what I do and congruent with how I do it, answering questions and feeling challenged is far less stressful. Furthermore, mistakes that happen in the course of following a routine with consistent and congruent professionalism are genuine, honest mistakes.

Communication is the hallmark of good, caring treatment. To ask permission, or at least acknowledge the normal, necessary boundary crossings as they happen provides safety for the practitioner and for the patient. Announcing yourself before entering the room is a courtesy, just as is saying, "I'm going to move your arm to take your blood pressure." By communicating in the process and regularly checking in with the patient, "Is this OK?" or "Is this comfortable?" the connection with the patient is fostered and improved. Maintaining a conversation about the procedure, whether it is a bed bath or a blood draw, keeps the patient open to expressing their fear or pain, rather than waiting until it is potentially harmful.

The other aspect of communication is asking for guidance. If something "feels out of sorts," whether it is with the patient or within myself, checking in with a peer, supervisor, or consultant is always the better course of valor even when I am not keen to admit that I don't know something or have made a mistake. In mental health practice, the adage goes, "Secrets keep us sick." One way to maintain internal congruence is to talk about questionable or difficult situations before they overwhelm us.

Part of maintaining boundaries is rooted in our **commitment**, first, to ourselves, then to our patients, and, ultimately, to the systems in which we work. Commitment to ourselves supports the consistency and communication necessary to set our individual professional goals and stay on course to meet those goals. In doing so, our internal congruence falls into place more easily. In addition, part of the commitment to ourselves involves "leaving work at work." That is, to talk through our problems during work hours, leaving time away from work for family, rejuvenation, and recreation in all their senses.

Next, commitment to our patients leads us along the path of doing not only what is "standard of care," but also doing the job with the kind of care, concern, and diligence that we would want to receive were the roles switched. Maintaining the boundary of doing what is best for the patient from all perspectives demonstrates our commitment to the patient.

Finally, the best measure of our commitment to the organization, institution, or system for which we work is our performance with the patients across all of these measures. Doing our best consistent, congruent job for each patient provides good patient care, greater patient satisfaction, and more congenial work environments.

Compassion is probably the most sensitive of the measures of appropriate behavior. Being overly compassionate can cloud our judgment just as much as being uncaring and dispassionate. Fortunately, the other criteria we have been discussing help with this process. By checking our consistency, congruence, and commitment, then asking for feedback and communicating, we are able to identify the appropriateness of our caring feelings. Rarely is it a failure of compassion to appropriately step back from the demands, needs, or wants of a patient. In fact, that sense of protest and wanting to distance from the patient may be a healthy countertransference in that the provider is resonating the frustration, anger, and many other negative feelings that the patient is having difficulty containing. This becomes a positive force in the therapeutic and healing process. When the provider is able to identify that he or she is setting a limit, it may very well help the patient understand how to define their own boundaries and where they need to stop.

The "Problem Patient" is Not the Issue

Many times, a first line of defense for someone accused of a sexual boundary violation is to accuse the victim of being seductive. Obviously, if the patient is incapacitated, too young or too old, or otherwise unable to protect him or herself during a sexual violation, all fingers point to the practitioner. Things become trickier with patient-practitioner or office romances, or in situations where the patient was the one exhibiting inappropriate behavior. In these cases, blame can bounce back and forth like a tennis ball. The patient or employee might have been the one to initiate the inappropriate behavior, but the practitioner is responsible for stopping it. The bottom line is that regardless of the patient's behavior, the responsibility for maintaining boundaries lies with the professional.

In our discussion of the power differentials in the provider-patient relationship, we emphasize that there are many levels at which power is transferred from the patient to the provider both consciously and subconsciously. In many of these cases, power cannot just be given back to the patient on their request. Once we enter into the professional relationship, we establish that power differential and it is our responsibility to redirect the seductive, sexually aggressive, or inappropriate patient.

While this may sound like a fairly straightforward and simple task, it rarely is. The many emotional and behavioral factors that lead a patient to be sexually aggressive with a provider are extremely difficult to understand and are rarely clearly verbalized by the patient. This is why, particularly in mental health, it is imperative that every practitioner understand that no therapeutic benefit comes out of sexual encounters between providers and patients. What may look comfortable and pleasant in terms of language and gestures may underneath involve layers of dysfunction and a painful history.

A further complicating factor in the practitioner-patient dynamic lies in the frequent mismatch between what the patient believes they need and what they ask for. For instance, a patient who was molested by an abusive parent as a child may seek the affection and acceptance of a caregiver. Because, historically, these feelings of affection and acceptance came in the form of sexual abuse, that is how they seek those feelings as adults. Conversely, the patient may interpret genuine care and affection from a practitioner as a request for erotic pleasure. Then, when that is not affirmed, the patient may react with rage and promptly file a complaint. That is one of the reasons why it is crucial for the provider to maintain boundaries for patients across the board. We never know how the patient interprets our gestures of kindness and, more importantly, how they may misinterpret them.

Redirecting Confusing Messages

Most of the time, interactions that may become seductive are preceded by confusing or mixed messages. Being on the lookout for messages that may have double meanings or that have extra beats of pause after them will help you identify potentially shaky boundaries. For example, increasingly personal questions that may appear benign, such as asking about children or family or where one lives, or comments about your appearance may be said with genuine concern or curiosity and have no underlying meaning. However, noticing these statements and redirecting the conversation to how the patient is feeling will help reinforce healthy boundaries. If a patient persists in making comments or asking personal questions, they may require firmer redirection.

Here are some steps that will be useful in verifying and responding to potentially inappropriate or seductive patients:

- **Never, never, never disregard your intuition.** Your intuition, inner sense, or "gut feeling" is based on many things that are both intellectual, physiological, and unconscious. Anytime you have a sense that what is going on is not quite right, trust that sense, but do not take it as truth engraved in stone. Remind yourself of your boundaries, and your duties during any encounter with the patient. Focus on these and continue to observe what your intuition tells you.

- **Discuss the interaction with your supervisor.** Any time you question an interaction with a patient, discussing it with your supervisor is wise. Simply laying out what was said, what happened, and how you felt, then asking for advice will lay the groundwork for further interventions, if they are necessary.

- **Directly and concisely redirect the patient.** Frequently, you will get the support of your supervisor to redirect a patient and request a change in their behavior. If done correctly, this support will focus less on changing the patient's behavior and more on helping you reinforce your boundaries. Simple statements such as "Talking about these things is not a part of my job." Or, "That is not an appropriate question for me to answer." Or, "I will be glad to get a person of your gender to help you with that." Simple redirection gives a clear message of where your boundary lies while making it clear that the problem is the question or the conversation. We don't want to shame the patient in the process. A dramatic reaction from the patient, such as feeling chastised, is probably an indication of more intense motives. Do your best not to react to their reaction and simply move on to the next topic or task.

- **Ask a peer or supervisor to join you on an encounter with a problematic patient.** If the advice given by your supervisor does not alleviate your discomfort, ask a peer or your supervisor to join you during an encounter with a problematic patient. Request that they observe the interaction for any evidence of what you have been seeing. After you leave the patient, review the encounter with them and ask for their feedback. If they have no feedback for you, keep in mind that the presence of another person in the room may change your behavior or that of the patient. Simply chalk it up to one objective opinion. Do not assume that you have been completely misreading the situation.

- **Consider requesting that that patient be transferred to another provider.** If your discomfort continues or if the patient continues to push against your boundaries, express concern to your supervisor or the person responsible for assigning patients and request that they should be moved to another provider. When making this request, be clear that you are not accusing the patient specifically, but that you are feeling uncomfortable and wish to stop any further problems before they escalate. Be sure to remind your supervisor of the type of patient you tend to do well with that other people may find difficult, such as patients who require physical strength or extra patience. In the end, removing sexually aggressive patients from your roster is a far better option than having to deal with the complaint that could potentially jeopardize one's license.

The power that practitioners gain in the patient-provider relationship should only be used for the benefit of the patient, and we can use that power to the greatest effect by maintaining appropriate boundaries. Though difficult, maintaining those boundaries is not only worth the effort, but, in the end, gratifying for us as individuals, the organizations for which we work, and for the patients who continue to gain the benefit of our services.

Patients' Rights

It is beyond the scope of this book to fully describe what victims should or should not do in the case of sexual misconduct by a physician or caregiver. Patients should always have the right to end an examination at any time they feel uncomfortable. They should always have the right to have a chaperone present in the examination or treatment room as well as a right to privacy. They should undress to a level of their comfort and be able to ask to be examined by a practitioner of a different gender. Before a practitioner touches a patient, he or she should answer all of the patient's questions and explain any procedures or examinations. Religious garments or jewelry should always be respected by the professional. You as the professional should not only recognize these basic patient rights but should encourage them. If a patient, supervisee, family member, or staff member experiences or witnesses abuse or assault, they should consider reporting the incident to law enforcement. The hospital, physician's office staff, or facility should be notified of the mistreatment or abuse, and the state's licensing board should be notified with a formal complaint.

Further Reading:

The American College of Obstetrics and Gynecology has an excellent opinion paper on sexual misconduct, developed by their Committee on Ethics, published online, December 19, 2019.

(https:/www.acog.org:Clinical-Guidance-and-Publications?Com, committee on ethic/sexual misconduct?)

Chapter 8:
Electronic Media: Positives and Negatives

"Do you grip your cell phone tighter than the hands of your loved ones?" –Rachel Stafford

Actress Rosemary Dewitt sums up electronic media and technology: "In some ways, technology has outpaced our ethics and the ability forever to understand the monster we have created. Technology is like a blender—it's just this inanimate object that does not have any feelings. It doesn't have a point of view. Its benign. It is just doing what we asked it to do, and that's the part we have to be careful of."

Social media is here and will continue to evolve as humans see fit. The numbers are staggering. As of 2018, there are 211 social media sites, but that number is sure to grow. There are 1.6 billion users of Google, 1.3 billion Facebook users, and 1.5 billion YouTube subscribers. Eighty-five percent of the world is connected by email or texts. There are 8.6 trillion interchanges per year, and for the most part, they are archived forever.[48] The most popular are Facebook, Twitter, LinkedIn, Flickr, Snapchat, Pinterest, Tumblr, Instagram, and CaringBridge. As with most technology, there are two sides to the coin. Electronic media is no different, so let's start with the many positive aspects and applications.

---

[48] Ventola, CL, Social Media and Health Care Professionals: Benefits, Risks, and Best Practices, PT, July 2014, 39 (7),491-499.

Social Media as a Tool

Social media has the power to help people connect to others whom they might not otherwise be able to connect. In healthcare, this is particularly helpful to physicians, as they can find experts or information that they need to do their jobs better. SERMO and Doximity are used entirely by physicians and other healthcare professionals. Both sites report over 800,000 users, which is a majority of the physicians practicing in the United States.

SERMO describes itself as a "virtual doctors' lounge" representing 90 specialties and subspecialties. There is a three-step credentialing process to assure physicians are communicating with fellow physicians. Ninety percent of SERMO users remain anonymous, possibly to make disclosing medical errors or lack of knowledge easier for the user. Crowd sourcing, case reports, clinical queries and advice, and medical education are all conducted through the platform. In 2016, users sought advice on over 7,300 challenging cases. SERMO also serves as the largest polling company for physicians and healthcare workers, allowing physicians to weigh in on medical issues, the business of medicine, and the stress and challenges of the profession.

Doximity is a Facebook-like social media platform for physicians and, for the most part, is not anonymous. A primary care physician can use Doximity to find a specialist for a patient. She can send and receive medical information through the platform to relay to a specialist. Providers can reach out to a potential colleague on the platform, but only after that interaction is accepted can the physician provide personal contact information. Doximity also has expanded into patient outreach by creating a smart phone app that allows physicians to call patients without revealing their phone numbers. Doximity reports that physicians, physician assistants, and nurse practitioners make more than 7,000 calls per day through the platform. Both Doximity and SERMO use the search engine platforms to target practitioners with advertising for medical drugs and/or devices.

In addition to these two independent healthcare-focused social media platforms, there are many social media platforms that are associated with institutions or that target specific specialties or demographics, such as students, international physicians, or female physicians. These internal or specialized social media platforms should be treated with the same care and consideration as the broader-reaching platforms, such as Facebook or Twitter.

Websites are the new "yellow pages." Every entity that is attempting to sell something or provide services has a website. Hospitals, group and individual practices, professional organizations, and specialty groups all have websites. There is no question that they are a powerful tool for building a brand, generating referrals, demonstrating a particular service or expertise, generating new patients, encouraging positive reviews, and educating the general public. For the most part, patients do not really care where you trained, whether you are board certified, or if you have a faculty position at an ivy league school. They just look at star ratings and reviews online.

Websites by themselves are not interactive; other than the risk of relaying misleading or untruthful information, engaging with a Website does not carry any real risks when it comes to boundary violations. If the website is constructed properly, with attention to issues regarding legality, ethics, and accuracy, then it serves the greater good. Imbedded YouTube videos put a personal touch to the effort as well, and if done professionally, can be a real plus. However, when you add an e-mail link and initiate a two-way conversation with the website user, then the risks arise. Many practitioners use a blog to generate interest or involve others in a conversation regarding particular topics. If comments are enabled on the blog, the blogger relinquishes control over how this conversation evolves. Inappropriate posts from readers that are inaccurate, rude, crude, or misleading must be addressed quickly. If it is on your site, then you own it. In addition, revealing patient health information through an online venue, either directly or indirectly, poses a huge threat to you and your practice.

Patient portals that allow patients to access their own medical information are gaining traction. Portals can increase patient participation in their own care. Through a secure portal, patients can access their lab results, radiographic interpretations, appointment history, upcoming appointments, medications, and visit summaries. Some portals allow the patient or client to exchange secure emails or texts with the healthcare team, mainly for appointments or prescription refills. There is a tether between the patient's personal health record and the hospital's or group's electronic health record. The security of this link is paramount to prevent exposure of the patient's personal medical history. Failure to protect this information can lead to Health Insurance Portability and

Accountability Act (HIPAA) violations. A secondary risk is that a patient will review his or her record and health information and make an uninformed decision without a healthcare provider's input. The concept and the technology have obvious benefits, but as the technology evolves, the ethical and legal risks need to be continually evaluated.

Telemedicine began decades ago to enable providers to exchange medical information with other medical professionals that were in remote or inaccessible sites. Radiographic and EKG interpretations were and still are used for those professionals who do not have ready access to such services. Today, telemedicine has become an industry unto itself. In 2016, telemedicine was a $30 billion industry and growing. NowClinic was organized in 2010 to provide online medical evaluation and treatment. A new patient can consult with a physician or nurse remotely. The signs and symptoms are relayed to the provider by email or texts, a diagnosis is made, and a prescription is emailed to the pharmacy, all for a fee of less than $50.00. A patient can access the site on their own or through their employer's or their personal health plan.

Pharmacies have also jumped on the telemedicine bandwagon. Many provide a small cubicle with a blood pressure cuff, a scale, a thermometer, and a lap top computer. The patient then clicks on the website, enters his or her credit card information or insurance information and has an "electronic appointment" with a healthcare provider. The provider makes a diagnosis, and the prescription is electronically sent to the pharmacist a few feet away. The benefits are apparent, but the legal and ethical risks are not.

It wasn't long before healthcare providers started adapting Skype and FaceTime to provide telemedicine. Some boutique medical practices offer Skype sessions. The promoted benefits of face-to-face patient contact allow the physician or nurse to see the patient—albeit via screen—for their evaluation. Although this type of telemedicine can be beneficial in a pinch, the potential for boundary violations here are enormous. People tend to lose some inhibitions when a screen is between them and the people they are interacting with. In addition, the session is not monitored, and there are no chaperones present.

Telepsychiatry is also an emerging trend. In a 2016 *Psychiatric News* article, Claire Zilban, MD, wrote: "Telepsychiatry uses a closed network established between two health facilities, such as an academic medical center and a rural clinic or correctional facility. It has enormous advantages for increasing access to expert care and includes built-in protections to safeguard confidentiality and uphold the standard of care." She states that Skype and similar technology can extend telemedicine to private practices and patients' homes, using technology that many people already have on their electronic devices. This is particularly helpful for patients who live in remote areas or have limited mobility.

Increasing access to care falls in line with APA's *Principles of Medical Ethics with Annotations Especially Applicable to Psychiatry*, which states, "A physician shall support access to medical care for all people." Zilban goes on to say that there are four major risks to this type of telemedicine: confidentiality, standard of care, safety, and regulatory compliance. Skype is encrypted but could be hacked. Non-professionals could be present outside the view of the camera, or the session could be recorded by either party without the consent of the other, which is illegal. Another challenge of using video-based media, particularly for psychiatry, is that a mental health assessment and subsequent care is more than just listening. Body language, voice inflections, tremors, skin flushing, etc. are all difficult to detect over the Internet. Telemedicine can connect patients and providers from all over the country, but the legal criteria require that the practitioner is licensed in the state in which he or she is providing care. FaceTime or Skype interactions with an established patient may have many benefits, but for new or unknown patients, take the time to consider the risks versus the benefits.

Pause Before You Post

There are many positives to the judicious use of social media in medicine, and the future will open many more possibilities. The risks, however, will not diminish in time; rather, the potholes will become bigger. Everyone, medical professional or not, would benefit from pausing before posting on social media. It has become too easy to type out a response, a rebuttal, an unkind or confidential comment, or an off-color joke and hit the "send" button. You cannot, as much as you try, separate your professional life from your personal life. Social media tends to fuse the two together. An in-person conversation may or will be lost, but a post, a blog, an email, a text, or a photograph may remain in the cloud forever. Before you hit "send," consider these questions: Is what I'm about to share legal? Is it ethical? Is it professional? Is it smart? Is it necessary?

Is it truthful and accurate? Are you comfortable with it being permanently associated with you? Anything you say or do on social media can come back to bite you.

A major risk of using social media is breaching patient confidentiality. Violating HIPAA can result in fines, censures, loss of license, and criminal actions. The law was written to allow healthcare providers and entities to share patients' healthcare information securely and confidentially with the consent of the patient. A healthcare provider (whether physician, nurse, physical therapist, or social worker, etc.) must be aware of how this law can be broken. An "innocent" post of a cute kid by a pediatric nurse, a clinical vignette on Doximity, or a photograph or video taken with a smart phone and made public via social media all violate the law. The law states that all personal identifying information and/or any revealing references must be removed. This de-identification can be accomplished by changing or omitting patient or client details, including names, social security numbers, hospital or insurance numbers, date of birth, or photographs. Describing rare medical conditions or occurrences within a specific time frame or location can also violate the law, as it may ultimately identify the patient. For example, an ENT surgeon posted on his Facebook page about his late-night visit to the local emergency room where he repaired a young girl's facial injuries sustained in a motor vehicle accident. He stated she was under the influence while driving. He did not post names or numbers, photographs, or other identifying information, but the location was rather isolated, and it was obvious to those who saw the young patient at school with the facial injuries that this was the patient he had treated. Her family sued on the basis of a HIPAA violation, and the case ended with a large settlement.

A study of medical blogs written by healthcare providers finds that of 271 samples, individual patients were described 47% of the time. Seventeen percent (17%) were found to include enough information for the patients to identify themselves or their providers. Three of the blogs included recognizable photographs of the patients[49]. The patient's consent is critical if their information is to be used in an article, a blog, or any other social media posting.

Most, if not all, organizations have policies and procedures concerning the use of social media both within the organization and outside of your professional role. Most healthcare professionals are not independent and answer to an employer and its human resources department. The HIPAA guidelines should be your guiding light, but the use of social media to disparage others, report petty or legitimate issues, air grievances, or promote your own agenda is inappropriate and will violate the institution's policies. Posts that are offensive, rude, or sexual in nature can be grounds for action or dismissal, whether done personally or professionally. Think twice before forwarding an inappropriate email or text. The thread will have your name attached indefinitely. A physician venting about hospital administrative procedures or a nurse or staff member accusing a physician of sexual harassment online would be grounds for dismissal. Again, pause before you post.

---

[49] Chretien, KC, Kind, T. Social Media and Clinical Care: ethical, professional and social implications. Circulation 2013, 1277, 1413-1421.

Posting updates to your social life online or via text or email can have significant repercussions. Medical staff service professionals routinely do a primary source verification of your licensure, education, and credentials. They do a criminal background check and assess the results of your drug screen. They also do a general internet search. Having a photograph on your Facebook page showing ten empty martini glasses in front of you while you are holding a weapon is probably not a good career move. Images of an overtly sexual nature is not in your best interest, either. A psychiatry resident's nude photographs were posted online by her husband without her knowledge. A fellow resident found the post and threatened to report her to the residency training program unless she agreed to have a sexual relationship with him. She declined, he turned her in, and SHE lost her position in the residency. Unintended consequences can be brutal.

Crossing or violating boundaries appears to be easier to do electronically. In the absence of a physical person with whom to interact, the normal social filters are removed. As discussed previously, there is a place for professional emails or texts in the care of a patient or in communicating with staff or subordinates. But it is important to treat the interchange the same as a face-to-face encounter. The power differential exists all the same. In many cases, the critical point where a typical interaction can flip to a boundary violation is between the exam table and the door. In other words, what you say or do once you have completed the professional interchange is critical. No follow-up text with heart or flower emojis lest you slide down a slippery slope. Many of the participants in our boundary courses began an affair online with a patient or a subordinate. The news media is overflowing with instances of boundary violations and sexual misconduct that began innocently with an extended online communication. Electronic and social media is here to stay and will continue to offer significant benefits for expediting information and communication in healthcare. But remember, anonymity is a myth; what you post, email, text, or blog is permanent and always traceable. You should protect your online presence as you would your professional presence. Pause before your post.

Take Aways
- Social media is both a blessing and a curse.
- Always pause before you post.
- Electronic media is permanent and retrievable and can be used against you.
- Always be aware of patient confidentiality when using electronic media.
- Protect your online presence by making wise decisions.

Chapter 9:
Long Term Strategies

Your ability to develop or maintain your professional boundaries as you embark or continue on your career in healthcare is predicated on knowing yourself. It is critical to understand the principles discussed in this book and to implement them within the context of your individual values and vulnerabilities. Many of us thought, when we attained our degree and license to practice independently, that we were bullet proof. One of my favorite quotes, which is unattributed, is "It is what you learn after you know it all that really counts."

If you are a licensed healthcare or mental health professional then you and you alone are responsible for your boundaries, and the best way to own that responsibility is by being honest with yourself and keeping checks on your personal emotional health. You must be honest with yourself about your vulnerabilities, triggers, and temptations. If you think what you are doing is wrong, even for a second, you are probably correct. Is the professional encounter centered on the patient's wellbeing or yours? Look in the mirror. It is important to accept that many of our boundary crossings are an aspect of normal human interaction, but they pose a slippery slope. Is hugging a patient always a bad idea? Is complimenting a person's attire a boundary violation? Is participating on social media an ethical breach? Of course not, at least not always.

One of the first steps to maintaining appropriate boundaries is developing your own emotional intelligence. Emotional Intelligence (EI) is a term first coined by psychologists John

Mayer and Peter Salovey in their 1990 book *Emotional Intelligence: Key Readings on the Mayer and Salovey Model.* The term, definition, and explanation have been expanded by several authors, but mainly by psychologist Daniel Goleman. In his book, *Emotional Intelligence: Why It Can Matter More Than IQ*, Goleman postulates that you cannot really alter your IQ, your genetics, or your family background, but you can alter and improve your emotional intelligence. In many ways, it may be more critical to success than your IQ.

EI encompasses several points. First and foremost is self-awareness, or knowing your own emotions. Knowing your feelings as they are happening, not after the fact or when someone confronts you, is the foundation for emotional intelligence. Secondly, managing your emotions based on your own self-awareness in real time is crucial. How you react to a circumstance or a person defines your human interactions, whether it takes the form of anger management or sexual attraction. Thirdly, the ability to self-control your emotions by delaying gratification and stifling impulses to accomplish both short- and long-term goals is a key to personal and professional maturity. Lastly, but possibly more importantly, EI involves the ability to recognize emotions in others (empathy), which is a primary people skill in any context. The good news is that all these facets of emotional intelligence can be taught and learned like any other skill.

Keeping stress and burnout at bay

We all have vulnerabilities, many of which we have no control over as illustrated in previous chapters. Our normal common-sense boundaries become porous at times of stress, burnout, or with personal and professional challenges. A divorce, a death of a spouse or close friend, medical malpractice litigation, employment uncertainty, etc. set us up to act or react in a way that we would not normally. Many times, we see a stable, highly functional professional betraying their own standards when their vulnerabilities are added to an ever-present list of stressors. When the professional succumbs to the pressure, he or she can become impaired. Impairment can be either physical or psychological, and it can lead to chemical or substance abuse. This cascading effect can result in a loss of your normal professional boundaries.

Professional burnout today, particularly in healthcare professionals, is the elephant in the room. The literature is copious and convincing that burnout is a real and serious problem. It is not a professional mental illness; rather, its genesis is lack of autonomy, systems breakdowns, and the sheer volume of work that healthcare professionals have to accomplish on a daily basis. Burnout is many times a precursor to boundary violations and impairments. It is beyond the scope of this chapter to fully develop this premise, but long-term strategies for self-care will help address the real possibility of burnout that more than 50% of health care professionals exhibit.

Some institutions are trying to prevent burnout by forming physician groups that meet once a month. They have a conversation about the virtues and challenges of being a physician. The organization pays for the meal and provides the venue. There is no agenda, no slides, and discussion leaders rotate. Sharing common concerns, fears, temptations, and self-doubt in a safe place without judgment has had a quantitative effect on decreasing burnout.

We are all vulnerable to impairments, which may include substance and alcohol abuse, burnout, depression, and the stress associated with caring for our fellow human beings. Living a balanced life can stop vulnerabilities from turning into violations. Most of the men and women we encounter with professional boundary issues exist in an unbalanced personal state. Balance can be viewed in several ways, but it is helpful to view it as a square divided in four, each portion occupying a quarter of the whole: Family and friends, recreation, spiritualism, and work. Start by acknowledging how you spend your time. Try making a pie chart of how you spend your time every day for several weeks, then look at the percentage of each activity. It is not realistic to apportion each of the four endeavors the same amount of time, but the closer you get to parity, the healthier you will be. If you notice that your first quadrant (family and friends) is looking bare, try spending more time with family and friends, particularly those who are not associated with work and who bring you joy. Your second quadrant, recreation, can be physical but does not have to be. It can be reading, painting, game playing, and so on. Your third quadrant (spiritualism) can be religious, but not necessarily. It is important to spend some time in solitude contemplating something or someone greater than yourself. This could be a daily quiet time of prayer, meditation, or a time of centering, just clearing your hard drive. Your fourth quadrant (work), will mostly likely be full to the brim. Consider your professional goals and whether they help or hinder your personal ones.

If balance is as difficult for you as it is for most of us, consider seeking out a mentor, life coach, or mental health professional to help you reach your goal of a more balanced life. It will pay huge dividends as well as decrease your vulnerability to impairments that can subsequently lead to boundary violations.

Professional strategies to keep boundaries in check

To frame this discussion, this book is directed at both the student and the experienced practitioner, as well as the practitioner who has had an allegation, board order, or suspension involving boundaries. Our boundary courses have been populated by licensed professionals who have been accused of boundary violations. Some involve sexual misconduct or sexual harassment involving a patient or staff member. Some forwarded an off-color joke or email. Some accessed a friend's personal health record without authorization. Some performed an operation on a family member. The list is endless. The following are some tips and strategies to help you keep your practice professional.

Consider physical space. Boundary crossings can take almost any shape. Just being physically too close to someone can be misinterpreted as a violation. Your body language, facial expressions, tone of voice, and eye contact (or lack thereof) speak volumes. Obviously, inappropriate comments or jokes about sex, sexual orientation, ethnicity, or religion are potential problems. Complimenting someone's attire can be a positive or a negative. Is it a fashion statement or a sexual comment? Is a hug appropriate? Who initiated it and why? Is it a frontal hug or a side hug? Does it last three seconds or ten? Who is witnessing it? Are the witnesses or the person receiving the hug uncomfortable? It's complicated. Maybe a pat on the forearm or shoulder would be just as effective as a gesture of your empathy and caring than a hug. Who thought a hug could be so complicated? Even a simple handshake in some cultures would be deemed inappropriate. Maybe we should just fist bump. The devil is always in the details. There are strong opinions on both sides, and the proper boundary for you may differ from your colleagues' and peers'.

Pause before you post. As stated in Chapter 8, the use of social media is a double-edged sword. It is a best practice to separate the personal from the professional. Avoid any crossover. Consider using different email addresses and phone/text numbers for communicating with your patients and clients than you use to contact friends and family. Don't "friend" your patients or your staff on social media. Be very cautious of forwarding emails, photos, comments, or jokes that might be considered offensive. Remember that even if you delete them, they are never really gone. Just because you are a licensed professional does not mean you cannot participate on social platforms, but it does mean you need to filter the content through a professional lens.

Beware gifts. Gifts from patients are always a puzzle. What if Bill Gates offers you his Rolex watch as a gift because he is grateful to you for providing him with exceptional care? Would you take it? The cost to him is inconsequential, but to you it is significant. What if a patient leaves a bouquet of roses at the front desk for you after her second office visit? What if a patient presents a watercolor he painted just for you? What do you do with the homemade pie or the bottle of Scotch during the holidays? What is the intent of the gift? Is it a thank you or a bribe for preferential care? Think about all this beforehand. Have an internal policy on how you will respond. How do you treat the mayor or the celebrity? Do they get special appointment times, do they get a private office visit before or after hours? Do you charge the same fee? Are your business relationships comingled with your professional relationships? How do you treat your friends, referral sources, or staff? All of these are examples of boundary crossings that can lead to outright boundary violations. Remember: it is not a problem until it is a problem.

Avoid mixing roles. Providing medical treatment to yourself, your immediate family, and your staff might seem like a good idea, but the urologist that performs his own vasectomy might not have the best surgeon or the best patient (It happens more than you think). The dentist who attempts to surgically remove his own mandibular third molar might have a difficult time explaining just why he thought this was a good idea. As stated by the Council on Ethical and Judicial Affairs of the AMA: "Physicians should generally not treat themselves or their immediate family." Not all physicians who self-medicate abuse medications, but many of those who abuse started by self-medicating. Forty percent to 75% of physicians in impaired physician programs were self-medicating at the time they were referred[50].

---

[50] PT Hughes, et al, *JAMA*, 1992:267

Like any other type of boundary violation, self-medicating is a slippery slope. It starts with a few meds to ease the pain after a fall, or maybe just a few pills to help get you through the overnight shift, but it can easily spiral out of control into addiction or even suicide. Male physicians commit suicide 1.4 to 2.3 times more than that of the general population, and female physicians commit suicide 2.5 to 4.0 more than the general population[51]. A study evaluating suicide in physicians revealed some sobering numbers. Of the 31, 636 suicides studied, 203 were physicians. There was no statistical difference in depression, substance or alcohol abuse, or known mental illness in either group. However, the toxicology in physicians revealed the use of benzodiazepines, antipsychotics, and barbiturates, but not anti-depressants[52]. Self-treating and prescribing are not isolated findings. Fifty-two percent to 90% of physicians admitted to self-prescribing, and 26% admitted to raiding the sample closet. Most were male and did not have a primary care physician[53]. Another study concluded that physicians have an increased percentage of mental health problems particularly related to burnout. Twenty-five percent of the physicians in a small study in New England admitted to treating themselves with psychotropic drugs within the last twelve months[54].

Treating family members, staff, students, or supervisees carries a similar risk. Treating or prescribing outside your

[51] LB Andrews, et al, Physician Suicide, Meds cape, 2012.
[52] K Gold, Gen Hosp Psych, Nov., 2012
[53] Christie, JAMA, 1998:280
[54] WE Mc Auliffe, et al, NEJM, 1986:315

specialty and outside of your office without proper documentation and charting is difficult to defend. Would you think a cardiothoracic surgeon performing coronary artery bypass grafting on their father or mother is out of line? Anecdotal conversations with many oral and maxillofacial surgeons defend their practice of surgically removing their own children's third molars under anesthesia in their office. Furthermore, they administered and prescribed controlled substances during and after the procedure. They violated state laws in most states by administering or prescribing controlled substances to a family member. Providing routine care for members of your staff is certainly expedient but mental health care, breast or genital examinations, or prescribing controlled substances may carry a risk greater than you want to assume. Of course, there are always exceptions. Emergency situations, like you're stuck in an elevator with a woman about to give birth, are an exception. Practicing in a small community where you are the only practitioner may not offer you an alternative. Always have a chaperone, always keep a complete medical record, always treat during regular office hours, and bill accordingly.

Keep professional relationships professional. Boundaries involving staff, either office staff or hospital or institutional staff, has always posed potential problems. Facetiously, if I were to ask how many physicians or nurses married their physician or nurse, many hands would go up. If I were to include second marriages, many more hands would go up. So, somewhere along the way for these folks, boundaries were crossed but not catastrophically. Again, it is not a problem until it is a problem. Sexual misconduct allegations to medical boards are commonplace when romantic relationships go south. It can take the form of whistle blower status, sex for drugs, surgical procedures for sex, sexual harassment, and so forth. The power differential becomes the key. It is best practice to have an office manual or human resource document that is patently clear. Your office manual should have a section detailing the definitions of sexual harassment and how it will be dealt with. It should be reviewed yearly by you and your staff and signed by all to ensure that everyone has read it and understands its meaning. Most people that work for you or that you work for sign the form because they want to, not because they have to. In other words, an employer-employee relationship should be a business relationship and not a social relationship. It is difficult to separate the two, but it is critical to acknowledge where you are in the equation. A written office policy can elaborate on hours, overtime, on-call responsibilities, OSHA regulations, HIPAA standards, and Equal Employment Opportunity Commission (EEOC) regulations, etc. Job description, compensation, and bonuses all should be discussed. Prohibition of salary advances and preferential treatment of some employees but not all should be included. Business trips, professional meetings, continuing education courses, also need to be addressed. It is beyond the scope of this book to cover all the contingencies, but your professional boundaries need to be protected whether you are an employer or an employee.

There are a few aspects you should consider that would probably not be codified in the manual. Your dating pool should not be your staff, either in the office or the institution. Avoid surrogate spousal relationships where you rely on your staff as primary sources of friendship or emotional support. It is helpful to understand your vulnerabilities, including your family of origin, attachment templates, stressors, etc. Out-of-town professional meetings with staff need to be structured. Special functions that include alcohol have been the basis for many sexual harassment allegations. Friday afternoon get-togethers or happy hours with staff to celebrate the end of the week with cocktails and chips is inadvisable. Holiday parties may have a place, but the venue and invitation list need to be considered.

A cardiothoracic surgeon was constantly asking out hospital staff personnel. He was single. They would turn him down, but after repeated efforts on his part, they would report him to human resources and the medical staff leadership. He would attempt to trade letting a student observe him performing heart surgery if she would agree to go out with him. When confronted with his unacceptable behavior, he emphatically stated "Well, do you want me to go to a bar to get dates?" The answer was yes.

Although this book has explored may types of boundary violations, it bears repeating that boundary violations are not always sexual in nature. Thoughts of treating the influential businesspeople with ideas of getting that insider trading tip is blurring the lines. Your ego telling you that you are the only professional that can treat this particular difficult patient or disease is a slippery slope. Francois Rabelats, a French satirist, may have said it best: "If you wish to avoid seeing a fool you must first break your mirror." The patient or the staff member who puts you on a pedestal—as good as it may feel to you—is not a healthy scenario. There are high-risk patients and high-risk staff members. Be aware of the cues, the comments, the body language. Listen to your staff or colleagues when they approach you with a warning about your behavior.

Always treat patients during the day during regular office hours with proper chaperones and proper documentation. Some specialties obviously would always adhere to this principle and others would not. Mental healthcare is not routinely provided with a chaperone, but most Ob-Gyn care is always done in the presence of another staff member. Don't disregard common sense. Most boundary violations begin when the patient is off the exam table on the way to the door. That is when the conversation turns personal. That brief time is the greatest risk to maintaining your boundaries.

Take-Aways
- Practice emotional intelligence.
- Be aware of your own vulnerabilities.
- Maintain and improve your life balances.
- Pay attention!
- Avoid mixing roles.
- Self-treatment is not a good idea.
- Get help. Do not go it alone.

Chapter 10:
Potholes and Pearls

This concluding chapter is written and designed for you to read periodically to refresh your memory on the key topics discussed in this book. An occasional skim through these bullet points may help you catch yourself before a boundary crossing becomes a boundary violation.

- Boundaries are mutually understood, unspoken physical and emotional limits of the professional relationship between the patient and physician or student or the supervisor and supervisee.
- It is often difficult to make a clear distinction between where the professionals' boundaries end and where the patient's or client's boundaries begin.
- Boundaries are fluid, rarely well-defined, and are nearly always situational and prone to misinterpretation.
- There are nonsexual boundary crossings and violations and sexual boundary crossings and violations. The former many times leads to the latter.
- Boundary crossings or violations are not a problem until they a problem, meaning that practitioners may knowingly or unknowingly "get away with" unprofessional behavior for some period of time before being reported and appropriately disciplined.
- In a practitioner-patient relationship, mutual consent does not exist because the patient is never in a position to consent. The innate power differential prevents the

patient/client/student from making a clear and appropriate decision.

- Vulnerability is a state many of us go to great lengths to avoid, but it can signal strength rather than weakness. It takes courage to say "I need help."
- You did not choose your parents, and you did not have a say in how you were nurtured as a child, but these both had a profound effect on your physician-patient relationships.
- Dysfunctional families produce dysfunctional adults.
- Your family of origin, personality characteristics, external stressors, addiction, compulsivity, and mental and physical illness can leave you vulnerable to boundary violations.
- A family history of addiction or undue religious or military legalism can lead to an unhealthy appreciation of boundaries.
- A chaotic, dysfunctional, or over enmeshed family may leave you unwittingly vulnerable to professional boundary violations.
- Attachment templates can be a key to how we act and react as adult professionals. Secure attachments provide a platform for normal psychological and social development.
- Earning a medical or any other professional degree does not necessarily make you an educated professional.
- The pressure of a professional education is Darwinian at times with an unhealthy tolerance for pressure and unreasonable expectations.

- The power differential takes on many forms: knowledge, communication, information, pain relief, experience, autonomy, perceived infallibility, and objectivity.
- The most important part of the provider-patient relationship is the power of trust that our patients place in us.
- Empathy is a necessary, meaningful, and critical skill to the delivery of compassionate healthcare.
- Empathy is a double-edged sword: too much can be a potential problem for the caregiver and too little is a potential problem for the patient.
- Medical professionals who communicate with appropriate levels of empathy have higher patient satisfaction rates as well as better clinical outcomes.
- Communicating empathetically increases the clinicians job satisfaction and reduces burnout.
- Central to good patient care is not only caring for patients but also caring about them.
- Empathy requires active listening. Patients respond to your body language, voice inflection, and eye contact more than your actual words.
- As the professional, you are responsible for the communication and its meaning.
- Many meaningful patient interactions involve boundary crossings, but remember boundaries are contextual and our humanity is critical to empathetic and effective care.

- Ethical behavior refers to the choices we make when no one else is looking, whether at home, in public, or in a practice setting.
- Ethical behavior hinges on multiple factors, including context, culture, professional standards, moral guidelines, family backgrounds and values, and religious beliefs.
- Ethical standards are not determined by the practitioner but by the fiduciary body that regulates and governs them.
- It if feels inappropriate, it probably is.
- The test of ethics should not be when confronted by temptation but by systematically educating ourselves on potential ethical traps.
- Poor boundaries invite harmful behaviors. The problem is rarely the issue.
- Problematic sexual behavior may require attention and treatment as in any other addictive behavior.
- Be vigilant when boundary crossings may lead to boundary violations. Nonsexual contact can progress to sexual contact without pretext.
- Healthy boundaries help define healthy sexuality and behavior. Consistency, congruence, communication, commitment, and compassion all play key roles in protecting and maintaining our professional boundaries.
- Never ever disregard your intuition. Discuss questionable interactions with a colleague or supervisor.

- You are not obligated to treat every patient. As difficult as it may seem, you can always tell the patient that their problem is greater than your ability to treat.
- Sexuality is in our DNA and affects every interaction we have as humans.
- Intimacy in a professional relationship is complicated. When sex is equated with intimacy, the concept of boundaries is moot.
- Your personal culture may determine how you view gender, sex, and power.
- Silence can speak volumes. Patients observe every gesture and facial expression in an effort to guess what is happening. They are always reading you.
- "Do you grip your cell phone tighter than the hands of your loved ones?" -Rachel Stafford
- Technology in many ways has outpaced our ethics and common sense.
- Safeguard your social media. It can be misinterpreted, distributed, or hacked, which can damage your personal and professional reputation.
- Pause before you post.
- Any content created on the internet is permanent. The cloud retains everything, and it can be used against you.
- Patient confidentiality is more at risk now than with simple paper records.
- It is what you learn after you know it all that really counts.

- Develop your EI. It may be far more important than your IQ, your degree, or your professional license.
- Our common-sense boundaries become porous in times of stress, burnout, or when we are challenged personally and professionally.
- Living a balanced life can prevent your vulnerabilities from turning into boundary violations.
- Avoid mixing roles: treating yourself, your family or even your staff can lead to unexpected boundary violations.
- Pay attention!
- Seek professional help. If you struggle, do not go it alone.
- Professional boundaries are gray, not black and white. It will be up to you, the professional, to determine what they should be for you. Listen to your internal chaperone. The challenge will always be to balance your humanity as a caregiver with the ethical risks of crossing your patient's boundaries.